The Miracle Diet

Like it or not, we're all on a diet, whether that includes eating a bag of chips or an apple. The only question is... are you on a diet that will make you and your family sick, or make you well?

The Miracle Diet

Lose Weight, Gain Health

10 Diet Skills

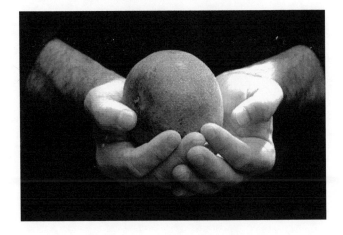

Susan Ford Collins

and

Rabbi Celso Cukierkorn

The Technology of Success

The Technology of Success
12040 NE 5th Avenue, Miami, FL 33161

Printed by CreateSpace
Cover design by Sharon Huff

This book can be purchased for business or promotional use and special sales.

To my daughters Cathy and Margaret and their amazing families!

To Albert, the other half of my heart and mind

Susan Ford Collins

To my beloved wife Jesse

and our beautiful daughter Sophie

Rabbi Celso Cukierkorn

Cover: The mango

Photo by: Susan Ford Collins

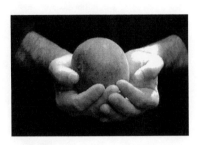

The mango is the most widely eaten fruit in the world. Sweet, juicy and delicious, mangoes are fat-free, sodium-free, cholesterol-free, high in vitamins and minerals and low in calories. Loaded with more than 20 vitamins and minerals, they defend the body against disease.

"Anyone wanting to lose weight will be sweet on mangoes. This versatile fruit is packed with nutrients, so you can eat less per meal and still meet the daily requirements for nutrition. Mangoes are also famous for their fleshy, stringy fruit, which is full of fiber and is a snack guaranteed to keep your raging appetite satiated until dinnertime."[1]

The Miracle Diet: Contents

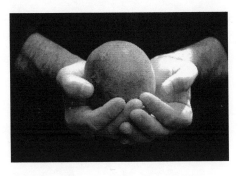

A secret Highly Successful People know... success has not one, but 3 essential parts!

Are you supersizing your body too?

75 pounds... the hidden inconvenience of convenience foods!

Bad food choices and a whole lot of denial. Does that sound familiar?

Beware, not all experts want what you want!

Experts 101... more than anyone ever taught you

23 gallons of fat! He drank 2,000 calories a day... before eating anything

Co-dreaders... don't let them kill your dreams!

Heads up... You're wired *not* to lose weight. Is wheat worse than sodas? Beware of The Addictive Mix!

Trick your body into burning fat!

What makes this diet book different?
Rabbi Celso Cukierkorn...

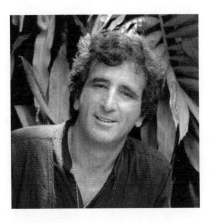

As a Rabbi, my job is to teach people how to enjoy more fulfilling lives. And to help them develop the discipline to care for their bodies, their families and our world. Yes, I was preaching it, but I wasn't doing it myself. And it was obvious.

All you had to do was look at me and you could see that I wasn't in control of *my body*. It would have taken a tent to cover up my belly! I had to be what I talked or my words wouldn't matter.

Somehow I had been able "to not notice" how much I was eating and the "100 pound impact" it was having on my body and my example to others... until one day something memorable and unexpected happened that changed everything.

I was on a plane heading home from Amsterdam when I heard the flight attendant shouting over the engine noise, "Please raise your hand if you requested a seat belt extender." She passed me twice because the obese man next to me was apparently too embarrassed to own up to his request. She handed it to him when he finally raised his hand, and I told myself a painful truth—

if I keep eating the way I am, I will soon be wearing a seat belt extender *myself*!

What had me stuck? Hadn't I noticed the clothes that no longer fit me being pushed to the sides of my closet? And my newer, larger ones filling in the center? Or the new belts I finally gave in and bought after punching as many holes in the old ones as I could? Hadn't I heard my doctor's advice to lose weight or else?

Yes, even in my food-induced fog I had noticed all that, but I had given myself excuses… like I'm heavy because of my genes, my dad was heavy, my brother is heavy. Or I'm not 20 anymore. Or I just don't have time to lose weight.

I bet some of this sounds familiar… you may also have felt as powerless as I did sitting at the table continuing to eat more and more, how comfortable (yes, sounds strange, comfortable!) I had become overeating and treating the acid reflux it produced in the night, or the apathy I had about making changes that would increase my time on this earth and the quality of my life in this body.

That day pointed out something essential I seemed to have forgotten… I know how to lose weight. *But I don' know how to keep that weight off!*

I had been on one diet after another and lost far more than 100 pounds collectively but I had gained it all back… and even more. What would it take for me to let go of the foods I knew I was addicted to? Or the habits that kept me stuck?

Clearly knowing *how to lose weight* and *how to maintain that weight loss* are two very different things! Lose, gain, lose, gain and lose again... an exercise in futility that no doubt sells lots of diet books but doesn't help people keep that weight off.

Imagining that seat belt extender locked across my body instead of his woke me up. From that moment on, I behaved differently. During the next layover I stopped in a restaurant and, instead of the thick creamy white dressing they were serving, I asked for oil and vinegar. Instead of letting them serve my meat covered in gravy, I asked for it on the side. Every three or four times I made even these simple changes, I lost a pound.

From that moment on, I saw losing weight and regaining my health as an essential part of *my work,* not something I could do *if* I had time and energy leftover. But something I needed to live and exemplify each day. Once my weight had become *my work,* it was much easier for me to lose those 100 pounds. The process was far more exciting than I could ever have imagined... especially watching my sizes drop, my belts shorten and the last 25 pounds melt away.

I had reached a new level... I wanted to learn *how to keep that weight off not just for a few weeks or months, but for the rest of my life.* Maintaining weight loss is a far greater challenge than losing it! I recently read that 99% of dieters fail to maintain their weight loss and, given my past experience, that statistic feels true to me!

Yoyo dieting had been my biggest weight loss challenge. I wanted to break that pattern once and for all. I would need an expert who could explain why the changes I made worked this time, what I had thought and done differently this time. Having reached my weight loss goal, I would need someone who could teach me how to manage old habits and familiar memories so they would not take over and make me fat again. I would need new skills.

I reached out to a nutritionist and a doctor and they both told me to simply continue eating the way I was. But I knew I wouldn't be able to do that without a new kind of support. They told me *what to do* but not *how to do it*.

Apparently God was invested in my renewal this time, because he immediately sent me the right person! The next day in an exercise class my instructor told me a new student, Susan Ford Collins, was a well-known author and success consultant and he asked if I was interested in meeting her. Not only did I meet her, but we worked out together. Standing side by side, Susan was amazed that I had lost 100 pounds. "Never in a million years would I have guessed that you had ever been heavy... no hanging skin, no sagging face, no indications at all that you had ever been anything but a trim, fit 40 year old!" Susan exclaimed.

We exchanged books and I told Susan I was writing a new book about weight loss, and I asked her to give me feedback when I finished my first draft. Once Susan read it, she challenged me to take this book much farther than I had.

To lose weight, *and keep it off,* you need 10 Diet Skills
"Diets fail," she said, "not because people don't know what and how much to eat, but because they lack the success skills needed to overcome the challenges of dieting long term."

I was stunned. It was like she had just read my mind!

Susan Ford Collins...

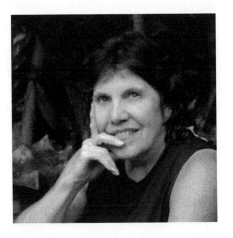

I read Susan's book *The Joy of Success* and learned that she had been helping top executives across the country do exactly what I wanted her to help me do. They could succeed themselves but they were unable to pass their success skills on to others in their organizations and families. By observing Highly Successful People (HSPs) for more than 20 years, she was able to discover *The Technology of Success...* the skill set it takes to make major long term changes in our jobs and our lives. In our weight and health.

Susan would wake me up, shake me up and make me aware again! Oh yes, I was resistant at first. I told myself I should be able to do this all by myself, but I knew I couldn't. I realized I had to set an example. To change, we have to reach out for assistance and be open to using it. No one of us knows everything. But all of us together know everything. Learning from each other is essential.

When I saw the power of what Susan had discovered, I asked if she would be willing to help me teach these success skills in *The Miracle Diet*. These skills will make this diet book stand out! They will teach you how to lose weight and keep it off for the rest of your life… for me, it has been over four years since I lost 100 pounds and I haven't gained any of that weight back! I am amazed at how this change has transformed my life.

Yes, I lost 100 pounds, but I didn't have a structure for organizing and teaching others what I had done. Life is like that. We do things, but we don't know precisely how we do them. I needed to know *how* so I could help you travel the path to long term weight loss and renewed health along with me.

Week after week, Susan pulled stories from me I hadn't remembered in years and pointed out exactly when and where I used each of the 10 success skills unconsciously. Their use was so obvious once she had shown me what I was doing and why, and it became far easier for me to use them again consciously. And teach them to you.

In addition, Susan and I will share information about food, diet and exercise you may not be aware of, information about additives and modifications food producers are making and how they are impacting you and your children. We will provide you with an overview of available diet plans and help you decide which ones might work best for you. As well as new information researchers are discovering that may be impacting your health now, or in the future.

The Miracle Diet... Three Miracles

First, you were given a *constantly-renewing body*. Second, *all the foods you need* have been provided. And third, you have a brain that is operating to coordinate your body and life *according to your instructions.* Unfortunately you have not understood the instructions you have been giving your brain so you have not always gotten the results you wanted. We are about to teach you the skills you will need to know *how* to fully enjoy these three miracles each and every day.

The First Miracle... your body is constantly renewing, if you know how to work with it

When you entered the material world, God lent you a body to act as a vessel and encase your soul. Your body is your temple and, miraculously, it is in a state of constant renewal.

Fat cells are replaced at the rate of 10% each year. Skin cells are renewed every two to four weeks. Your 9,000 taste buds are renewed every 10-14 days. Your skeleton is renewed every two years. Every day billions of cells replace the ones that came before them. You are in this miracle of creation and renewal every second of your life... unless you mess up that renewal.

God not only gave you a constantly renewing body, but he also provided a profoundly rich, diverse and constantly-renewing food supply.

The Second Miracle... you have been given the perfect foods

God provided all the foods, vitamins and minerals you need to be healthy. Squashes, beans and leafy greens. Grains, seeds and roots. Grapes, apples and pears. Pineapple, rambutan and jaboticaba. Oils, nuts and fibers. We live on a planet that grows all the foods we need in the area where we live. All the fish and meats. A diverse planet filled with various landscapes... lakes, rivers and oceans, plains, valleys and mountains. Various temperatures and humidities, tropics and deserts, constantly changing seasons and harvests.

The Third Miracle... you have been given the most sophisticated computer in the world

God has given you your own internal computer that monitors your temperature, your water level, your energy level, your organs and hormones, your healing and renewal, whether you are awake or asleep. All this is done for you unconsciously but there are parts of your brain that you need to learn how to operate consciously. Unfortunately, no one has ever explained your role in operating this computer so you have made errors and received error messages you haven't known how to use to make corrections. In this book we will teach you the basics of a conscious life.

It is not just what you eat and the amount of exercise you do that has you *stuck* at your current weight, it's also what you think. Here is a truth we will prove later on. *What you think is what you get... like it or not.*

If you learn *how* to manage your mind and stay focused and confident, then you can renew your body and your ability to experience a healthy fulfilling life.

Let me continue telling my story

When I was approaching 40, I realized that my father had his first heart attack at my age. Sadly Dad died from complications of diabetes, losing toe after toe, then his foot and leg at the knee.

Both of these devastating health conditions, heart disease and diabetes, are weight-related and manageable even though our family didn't realize it at the time. My father was not able to be at my wedding, but I want to make sure I am alive and well at my daughter's wedding.

Almost 40 and 100 pounds overweight, I had a vital decision to make. Would I continue pursuing "my father's dying process," or would I cooperate with my constantly renewing body and finally learn how to take care of it?

Today, 100 pounds lighter, I know renewal is possible. I have been able to transform my body and my life. Today I weigh less than I did when I was 21. I have more strength, muscle and vitality and a tremendous zest for life. Using *The Miracle Diet* approach, I have regained a healthy, lean, well-defined body... the body I want... and the life I want to live. And you can do this too.

Here are my before and after pictures.

Soon you will be marveling at yours.

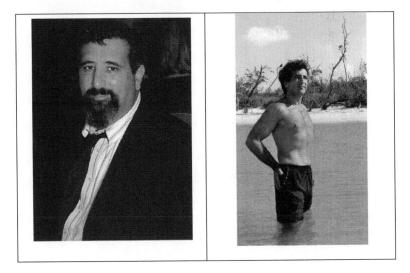

For three years, my weight has remained the same but my sizes have continued to drop. I lost *over one-third of my body mass and replaced it with lean muscle* which continues to burn body fat even as I sleep!

Remember, you are not a heavy person trying to slim down. You are a trim, healthy person learning how to reemerge.

Today's reality... we're fat and getting fatter!

We're fat and getting fatter... at great cost. According to the *American Journal of Preventive Medicine,* by 2030 42% of people in the United States will be obese or roughly 30 pounds over a healthy weight. Of those 42%, 11% will be severely obese... 100 pounds or more overweight.

We haven't yet reached 2030, but already by 2010, 36% of American adults were obese. And 6% were severely obese.

If the obesity rate continues to increase as predicted, and there's no reason to think it won't, we could have more than 100 million obese people in the U.S. *within just 18 years*. These numbers are staggering and they come with a huge price tag.

The *American Journal of Preventive Medicine* report says this increase in obesity would cost an additional $550 billion in medical expenditures between now and 2030. Meanwhile, one *out of every three children in the United States is currently obese or overweight.*

Carrying around all that fat (sometimes as much as 23 gallons of it) increases your risk for diabetes, heart disease, sleep apnea and several types of cancer, not to mention a shorter life expectancy, physical pain and limitations.

The reason people fail to lose weight usually isn't because they lack a good diet plan, but because they don't have the success skills to carry that plan through. Most diet books do a great job of telling you what to eat and how much of it to eat, but they fail to prepare you for dealing with the internal resistance that diets create, the old memories and past failures, the procrastinations and excuses. Your inner enemies. They also fail to prepare you for the external resistance, the disagreement and negative input that will start coming your way *as soon as you proclaim you're on a diet*. Your unexpected outer enemies.

Diet Skill One: Success Filing... when your Success File is full, you feel Success-Full

I was curious. I wanted to know whether... like the Highly Successful People (HSPs) Susan had been observing... I had been using all 10 success skills. If I had, I wanted to know precisely when and where I had used each skill so I went to see her.

Why are some people far more successful at weight loss... and everything else?

It was 10 am as I pulled into the semi-circular driveway in front of Susan's sprawling, tropical, Old Florida home. As she walked toward me with a warm smile, her gentle dog Honey greeted me too.

Susan's home is large, open and bright, with floor-to-ceiling windows overlooking a lush, sparkling Koi pond. We strolled down a long sunlit hallway past palms, orchids and bromeliads, by treasures Susan had collected from all over the world, and settled down on comfortable brown leather couches in her office.

"Welcome Rabbi," smiled Susan. "Before we start, there's just one thing. As we begin, you will need to set aside the rabbi part of you... the part of you that graduated from rabbinical college, who was a rabbi with his own temple and congregation, who traveled the world speaking to large audiences and who has written bestsellers. That isn't the part of you I will be coaching now.

The part I will be coaching is the fearful part, the compliant part. The part that is frustrated and confused. He's the one I will be teaching and encouraging. And with your permission, he's the one I would like to call Celso.

This is important, Celso, because we unconsciously feel we should be as smart and well-informed in all areas of our lives as we are in our areas of expertise. But we're not. So automatically feeling that we have to say *Yes, I know* can block learning. This applies whether you're a rabbi, a teacher, a lawyer, a doctor, a parent or a friend. *Being willing to not know* opens the gate to change," added Susan.

For a moment, I felt stripped of my rabbinical authority, but I knew Susan was right. Rabbi wasn't the part of me who just stepped through her door. And rabbi isn't the part of me who feels scared and insecure as I approach this new challenge. So I quickly said Yes, call me Celso and we began.

When did your weight problem begin?

I was a skinny kid growing up in Brazil. I rarely finished all the food on my plate. My parents frequently stood over me and delivered their "starving children in Africa" speech. Fortunately I knew that eating everything on my plate wouldn't help those kids.

To make sure I consumed enough calories, my family's cook made dark chocolate cakes full of sugar and farm fresh butter, especially for me. Ironically my brother was heavy and always on a diet so our parents were constantly telling my brother *what not to eat* and telling me that I *needed to eat more*.

As long as I finished my meat and vegetables, I could eat as much cake as I wanted. I was playing sports at school and ping pong and tennis at home so I didn't gain weight. But when I reached my 30's, I started putting on a couple of pounds a year.

When Jesse and I first married, we ate at home a lot. Jesse is a wonderful cook. But when our daughter was born and Jesse was finishing her Ph.D., eating out became the norm. As a rabbi in a university town, my job kept me busy. My responsibilities kept growing… and so did I!

I rushed from coffee meeting to lunch meeting, from dinner at a congregant's house to teaching adult education classes long into the evening. Food was served everywhere. I was offered appetizers and fat-filled foods plus coffee and desserts at each stop. It would have been rude to refuse what my congregants were offering me, wouldn't it?

Susan immediately zeroed in on the word *rude*. "Celso, did you hear what you just said? Rude to refuse! That's an old part of you speaking, a part that was taught to feel guilty about saying No to parents and teachers, to grown-ups in general when you were a child. But at this point in your life, *not saying No to others is saying No to your health and dreams.* This is just one of many old beliefs that are blocking you and need to be updated. We will discover more unconscious limits as we continue working together.

Today we will begin building the self-confidence you will need to say No to temptations, whether from your congregants, your family or others, No to old ideas and weight-gaining habits.

You probably thought we would start off talking about calories and fats, menus and recipes. That's what you have always done before, isn't it? How many diets have you and others you know been on? *Weight Watchers, Atkins, The Zone, South Beach* or Kate Middleton's favorite, the *Dukan Diet*.

Most diets work *if you are able to work them, but most people can't.* Their weight yo-yos up and down and their health and self-confidence yo-yos up and down with it."

Susan handed me a stack of lined pages numbered 1 to 200 and told me I would have 20 minutes to jot down 200 successes. That shouldn't be hard, Celso. They can be successes from *anytime in your life."* Then she set a timer and left the room and I started writing.

When Susan came back and saw me sitting there on her brown leather couch, chewing on my pen with only 20 successes on my list... only 20 successes from my whole life... she asked this all-important question. *"As you scanned your memory, Celso, what were you searching for?"*

Hmm, I've never really thought about how I define *success.* I guess its accomplishing things, getting good grades, passing exams, earning degrees, getting married, buying a home and developing my career.

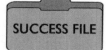

SUCCESS FILE

Reader: Before you any go farther, turn to your Success File in the back of the book. The lines are already numbered so you can do this vital exercise too. Or you can write them on lined paper or start a computer Success File to hold your successes for you.

Your new best friend... your Success File

"Well Celso, just so you know, the number you listed is almost exactly the same number of successes that participants in my *Technology of Success* seminars listed," Susan added. "They usually included getting good grades, being chosen for a team, making the honor roll, graduating from high school, being accepted to college, buying your first car, meeting and marrying, having your first child, buying your first home, receiving honors, awards, promotions and bonuses.

But 20 successes *for your whole life* is far from the truth! And far below the number of successes you will need to succeed at *any* diet or exercise program. Or *any* change you want to make in your life. That number simply tells me that your definition of success is off. Really off! We have some work to do before we talk about shopping lists, calories, sodium, sugar and fat. We need to begin exploring what makes you feel successful and confident, and what negative forces send you off in the wrong direction."

The first skill is Success Filing

Susan spent 20 years observing Highly Successful People (HSPs) for months at a time, driving to and from work with them, going to meetings with them, following them around when things were working well and when they were going crazy.

"I noticed that HSPs regularly stopped for a few minutes between appointments or in the car *to mentally rewind their day and review their realizations and accomplishments,*" said Susan.

"They asked themselves... Did I wake up with a good idea? What was it? What did I do next? Brush my teeth. Take my vitamins. Eat a good breakfast. Go for a walk or run. Take out the trash. Check

17

mail, email or phone messages. Reschedule meetings. Update my priorities. Review spelling words with my child on the drive to school. Stop to pick up dry cleaning and cash at the bank. Buy high-quality cold cuts, fruit or a salad for lunch, healthy food for dinner.

I watched HSPs repeating these words like a mantra. *I told myself I would and I did. I told myself I would and I did.* They were accountable to themselves. And they were accountable to others.

Instead of needing *other people to acknowledge them*, they had learned to *acknowledge themselves* for their all important business decisions and presentations, as well as their personal achievements as spouses and parents. They were very clear that *all these successes were what made their lives and careers work... success-fully."*

Every little success counts

This is the first success skill Susan observed HSPs using consistently, even though they didn't realize it until she pointed it out to them. This daily review process is what she calls *Success Filing*.

"Most people spend time at the end of each day thinking about all the things *they didn't get done*. All the things they *failed* to do. HSPs did that of course, but they spent much more time noticing *what they did get done*, what they accomplished.

Unlike my original HSPs, when I told others I coached about Success Filing, they frequently scratched their heads dubiously saying, 'But I felt these small, everyday successes didn't count.' To which I responded emphatically, "No! These usually "too-small-to-notice successes" absolutely do count and they are absolutely worth acknowledging. In fact, they are what we spend our days doing. These small successes accumulate into big deals and promotions, happy relationships and families. You can't get there without them. It's kind of like trying to jump the Grand Canyon instead of climbing down one side step-by-step and then climbing back up the other side step-by-step.

Imagine how you'd feel if you forgot to buy gas and arrived late for a meeting *you were leading*. Or if you were late to pick up your child and she was left alone and afraid. Or you promised your spouse or friend you would go out to dinner and a movie and you totally forgot. Or you promised your son you'd come to the baseball game he was pitching and you didn't show. Clearly these small successes... remembering to buy gas, picking up your child on time, keeping commitments with friends, and cheering your son on at his baseball game as promised... count. And count big!" she exclaimed.

Susan encourages business owners, managers and executives she coaches to not just Success File for themselves but to ask their employees to Success File as well. And to encourage their employees to share some of their successes with them so they can acknowledge actions they are taking, not just toward work goals, but toward health and balance goals as well.

When it comes to diet and exercise, every little success counts. Eating breakfast. Packing your lunch and your kids' lunches. Planning your day's food. Shopping for lean chicken, beef or fish, fresh fruits and vegetables. Having healthy snacks with you wherever you go. Keeping nuts in your pocket. Drinking plenty of water. Saying No to birthday cakes and pizza at work. Passing the vending machine. Eating an apple instead of an apple strudel.

Packing your workout clothes and shoes, and putting them in your car for later. Taking your towel and water bottle with you.

These 200 Successes are just the beginning. By the time you finish reading this book, you will have thousands of other successes you can add to your Success File. Your loose pants. The new hole in your belt. The smaller-size shirt you just bought. The compliments you're receiving. The way you feel when you catch sight of yourself in a mirror or plate glass window. Your new understandings about food and exercise. So you might want to buy a blank, lined notebook to use as your Success File. Pick one you really like, one that feels as special to you as your successes will.

What kind of confident are you? Other-confident or self-confident?

Reliving your successes will give you the strength to say No when you are tempted to eat that last piece of apple pie on the plate, or those chocolate chip cookies you're being offered with such a warm, lovely smile. Or when you want to blow off your exercise class or skip your workout because you are stressed or tired. Remembering the thousands of successes you've already had will empower you to continue losing weight and gaining health.

Most people don't like the word diet

Like it or not, we're all on a diet! Whether your diet includes eating a bag of Oreos or an apple, you're always on a diet. The only question is, are you on a diet that will make you live or make you die?

You must change your mind to change your weight

"You could have all the right foods in your refrigerator or on your menu and still not eat them. You could know what you should eat and still not eat it. *You've got to change your mind to change your weight and your health.*

There will be challenges ahead and, unlike most dieters, we want you to be confidently-prepared to say NO. Or, if you have already said yes and eaten that apple pie or those chocolate chip cookies, whether by bad-choice or by bad-habit, you will have the self-confidence to say NO next time and get right back on track.

Here's an important phrase to remember...
When your Success File is full, you feel success-full.
When your Success File is low, you feel dependent and needy.
And needing food too!

Success can be elusive as you will soon see, Celso. That's why you were only able to recall 20 successes *in your whole life!* Hard to believe, isn't it? But there are important and revealing reasons why.

More about success... what it is and what it isn't
According to *The New Webster's Dictionary*, success is the accomplishment of what is desired or aimed at.

So Celso, your definition of success lines up with Webster's. But *not with the definition of success HSPs used!*

Most people don't know realize that success has not just one, but three essential parts

For HSPs, accomplishing goals *is just one part of success.* They understand that Success has *three* essential parts:

1-Success is completion
2-Success is deletion... and
3-Success is creation/re-creation

Success is the ability to complete the tasks and goals you have in mind and others have in mind for you.

Success is also the ability to delete ideas and approaches that no longer work for you. Old habits like telling yourself you're too tired or too busy to take care of yourself. To eat right and exercise. Old dreams that were never yours in the first place. That were your parents' or teachers' or society's dreams *for you*.

Success is also being able to create new plans and dreams, big juicy exciting dreams that make you eager to wake up and take action. And success is being able to delete and recreate them along the way," added Susan.

*Reader: Let's take a few minutes to think of some completion, deletion and creation/recreation successes you have had since you woke up. Like eating a good breakfast or going for walk or putting out the trash. Or parking at the far end of the lot and walking to the building.

Success in your past, gives you confidence in your future

The word *confidence* comes from the Latin *confidere*, to have faith in. And in this case, it's faith in your ability to create the slimmer, healthier you. In my case, it's faith in being able to dance at my daughter's wedding!

A common diet mistake you don't want to make!

"Most people on a diet or exercise plan define *success* as *losing weight*. When they don't lose weight that day or that week, they tell themselves they've failed and slip back into their familiar failure cycle. I can't. This just doesn't work for me. I give up. Or I've already blown it. What the heck, I'll eat the rest of the cookies in the box. Or the potato chips in the bag. Or the ice cream in the freezer. Or I'll eat that last slice of pizza!

Daily Success Filing will keep you out of the *I didn't lose weight today so I failed trap* that keeps millions of Americans stuck in yo-yo diets, obesity and weight-related diseases.

When your Success File and your self-confidence are low, there is probably a "failure food" you crave. Salty, sweet, crunchy, carby or fatty? Which is yours? Most importantly, where do you usually go to get that food? That is probably a place you will want to avoid until you are well on your way to success. Staying away from temptation is a very good strategy. Another important question is, *who* do you pig out with, and when? Who do you drink with, and how much?

Self-confidence... the "winning ingredient" most diet books leave out

Success can't mean losing weight every day! That just isn't the way weight loss/health gain works. There will be plenty of days when you won't lose. Success on those days is continuing to eat and exercise *as planned*. Success is noticing all the small successes you are having that will soon change the number on the scale. And your cholesterol, blood pressure and blood sugar numbers as well.

Knowing how to build and rebuild your self-confidence is 'the winning ingredient' most diet books leave out. So before you rush out to buy the right food or sign up for an exercise class, let's slow down a bit and make sure *you are ready and able*. Let's do losing weight differently... successfully... this time.

What kind of confident are you? Other-confident or self-confident?

When you were a child, you were taught to have confidence in others... parents, teachers and adults. Confidence in what they knew and wanted you to do step-by-step. Given your immature body and huge lack of experience, putting your confidence in them was a smart approach.

Your parents and teachers made time to acknowledge the successes you were having... *from their point of view*. They wanted to be sure YOU knew what THEY wanted you to do, the way THEY wanted YOU to do it.

They taught you to feel the way they felt about your successes. When you learned to talk, they were thrilled. And so were you. When you learned to walk, they clapped their hands. And so did you. When you learned to write, read and do math, they gave stars, good grades and extra privileges. And you loved getting them. When you spoke publicly, they honored you with special ceremonies and celebrations. They felt proud of you and so you felt proud of yourself.

In your early years, your parents, teachers and society did your Success Filing for you... the same way you are doing it for *your* children. That's the reason you remembered the successes you did. Those were the successes THEY had in mind for you. The successes THEY acknowledged and celebrated with you... getting good grades, making the honor roll, graduating from high school, getting into college, getting married and having a child... you remember the list," chuckled Susan.

My artistic success was a failure in my father's eyes

Now that I am a parent, I can see that I wasn't easy to parent, or easy to acknowledge either for that matter. Imagine this.

As a teenager I was a creative painter, so creative in fact that I spray painted a brightly-colored mural on a huge wall near our home. My work of art was quite large and I painted it in broad daylight with lots of people walking by, so of course I was caught. My father received a phone call providing him with all the vivid details.

No, my father didn't acknowledge that creative success. Hardly. He saw it as a gigantic failure. He was the one who had to apologize to our neighbors and pay to have their wall cleaned and repainted. Even though my father was upset, I loved what I had produced. I wish I had a picture of that mural today. I can still see it in my mind. A brilliant beginning but unfortunately I have never done any murals since. Or any artwork for that matter. Despite this, I did learn something important from that early failure. The next time I paint a precious work of art on somebody's wall, I will ask their permission first so they will be excited too, and so my mural won't be painted over.

My father failed to recognize my creative success, but there's a far bigger question for me to consider. Did I unconsciously agree with my father's failure label? Is that why I never produced another large mural or any other artwork for that matter? What else did he disagree with that I have not done since? How might *his limits* have *limited me*… unconsciously?

"To change your life and your world, you can no longer depend on other people to Success File *for you*. HSPs understand that if you continue to rely on others for acknowledgment, you will have to keep doing what THEY want you to do, the way THEY want you to do it.

Success Filing... acknowledging yourself lets you choose

To succeed at anything that is uniquely your own, you will have to assume responsibility (response-ability, the ability to respond) for acknowledging yourself. Why? Because your new idea has never been done before, it will be seen as impossible to others. It will be disagreed with! Ask Bill Gates or Jeff Bezos or anybody else who has broken through the impossible to the possible. Remember, Jeff Bezos sold his home and all his possessions and relocated his family to start his, what seemed at the time, unlikely dream... amazon.com. You can only imagine how much disagreement he stirred up.

Innovators and inventors, business entrepreneurs and artists around the world have told me repeatedly that their friends and family-- the people from whom they most wanted support and enthusiasm-- were upset when they headed off in their new direction. They were mad, sad and disappointed. To try to prevent these innovators from proceeding any further, they made discouraging remarks or told them about individuals they knew who had failed at what they wanted to do... potentially poisoning their minds and draining their self-confidence.

Maybe you have had the same experience. Instead of *dreaming with you*, your friends and family *tried to discourage you*," observed Susan.

My aunt from Uruguay

When I started my diet and excitedly shared with my family that I had lost my first 10 pounds, my aunt responded, One time I lost 10 pounds and I gained it all back in a month.

When I lost 20 pounds and shared my excitement with my family, I didn't remember what my aunt had told me before. But this time she replied, one time I lost 20 pounds and then I gained back 25!

"Celso, this sort of negative reaction was disappointing to say the least, but there may have been a far greater disappointment than anyone in your family realized at the time. Instead of continuing to share your goals and dreams with your family, you probably stopped telling them anything at all. What a terrible loss for them, and for you.

Why saying NO is so hard to do

Not saying No to others is an old habit with deep emotional roots. Saying No in childhood led to disapproval and having things taken away... food, freedom, privileges, TV or the car. Saying No frequently meant you were a failure in others' eyes. That hurt and so you were afraid to say it," observed Susan.

The hardest No. The best fruit salad

Each year during Passover, I visit a couple in their late 80s. I bring them a box that contains everything they need to celebrate the holiday, matzah, horseradish, turkey breast, gefilte fish, parsley and a shank bone. Leah is a Holocaust survivor who spent so many years close to starvation in a concentration camp that she lost her ability to give birth to a child. Each year I visit Leah and Jacob in honor of the children they could never have.

The first time I visited their home after starting my diet, they offered me a babka, a sweet yeast cake that was definitely not on my diet or even close to it. It was time for me to figure out how to say No, and say No in a way they could understand and support. And so I began. I'm sorry, my dear friend, but I'm on a diet. Immediately she responded but eating is a blessing. I acknowledged that eating is a blessing but at this point in my life, *overeating is a curse*. It could be the end of me!

Leah said she understood (especially when I pointed to my large belly) but she still wanted to offer me something to eat whenever he came to their home. What can I make for you? How about a fruit salad? From that moment on, whenever I visit them, we share the blessing of food with coffee and fruit salad. They feel successful and so do I.

It's not about No. It's about how you say No

Thank them first, then request. Share your goal and make them codreamers.

Loving with food can be a serial killer

According to the Centers for Disease Control and Prevention (CDC), overeating is the most well-known and widespread killer in the U.S. For adults and now for teens.

According to the CDC, between 1999 and 2008, the percentage of adolescents ages 12 to 19 who have diabetes or prediabetes increased from 9 percent to 23 percent. Prediabetic blood sugar levels are abnormally high but not high enough to be classified as diabetes. The study also found that 50 percent of overweight teens and 60 percent of obese teens had at least one risk factor for cardiovascular disease.

Are we passing our weight and health problems on to the next generation? Isn't it time to set a healthier example? *Our Children Are Watching* is the title of one of Susan's other books. Yes, our children are watching and they are copying the way we live our lives, what we eat and how we exercise. Will our failures come back to haunt our children in the future? Or can we turn this problem around now, for us and for them?

If your scale bothers you, throw it out

Large successes, like losing 10 pounds or a 100, are made up of thousands of small successes like eating an apple instead of downing a soda. Making a list before you shop. Reading menus and labels carefully before you buy and consume. Doing what you tell yourself you'll do instead of procrastinating or making excuses and letting yourself down.

Losing weight doesn't happen on the scale. So if compulsively watching your weight move up and down distracts you, put your scale away. Stay on your plan and bring your scale out in two weeks or a month. Or weigh once a week at about the same time.

Some people gain weight when they begin exercising and building muscle. This is not a long term problem. Your weight will level out. Losing weight/gaining health is a marathon, not a sprint! It took me a year to lose 100 pounds, that's about two pounds a week. Some weeks I lost nothing. Some weeks I lost six pounds. For the past three years, I have built lean muscle with no major weight change, but my sizes have changed. When I started dieting, I wore size 42 pants. After one year, I was in a 34. Right now, after muscle building, I'm in a 30. And my weight has stayed the same.

Moving out and living away from your parents

"When you went off to college or found a job and moved into your own place, your parents were happy but a bit worried... worried about what you would do without them. Without their confidence and direction. Without their knowledge and acknowledgment.

Little by little your life and your parents' lives headed in different directions. They knew less and less about your life and your successes. They weren't there to acknowledge you, and you may not have been prepared to acknowledge yourself.

Chances are good that during childhood, no one ever sat down to explain success and self-confidence to you the way we just did. They didn't teach you what *success* is and how to recognize all three essential parts, *completion, deletion and creation*. And they didn't teach you how to Success File because they didn't Success File themselves. Therefore *when you were alone for the first time, and you most needed your own confidence-building skills*, you simply didn't have them."

Susan has coached first year college students who could easily do the new course work, but who couldn't build enough self-confidence to compete at this new level. A number of colleges sit freshmen down in the auditorium their first day. "Look to the right of you and look to the left of you. Those students were at the top of their class too and that's who you will be competing with. You'll be a little fish in a big ocean from now on." Susan remembers that speech well from her first day at Smith College.

As we begin *The Miracle Diet*, we are teaching you how to Success File so this time you will have the self-confidence skills you need to stand up to conflicting ideas and opinions, conflicting goals and dreams. So this time you can stay on course in "the big ocean of weight loss/health gain."

Good boy or healthy man?

"Celso, not saying No" to your parents may have made you a good son," smiled Susan. "*But not saying No* to congregants offering you cakes and cookies at weddings and Bar Mitzvahs was causing a dangerous health problem... Severe Obesity, carrying around 100 pounds or more of extra weight.

The health problems associated with being overweight go way beyond heart disease and diabetes. Being overweight can also affect your joints, breathing, sleep, mood and energy levels. Being overweight impacts your quality of life, and the quality of life of the people you love.

It's time to remember this vitally important fact. Yes, *vital* because *your life literally depends on it*! *Saying yes to others* sometimes means *saying No to yourself*, to your goals and dreams, to eating and exercising the way you need to in order to lose weight and gain health. Continuing to depend on others to acknowledge you may mean you will lack the self-confidence to say YES to yourself. To stand your own ground.

No is your protective fence

The word No lets you set limits. Other people may be disappointed to hear your Nos at first, but once you share your weight loss goals, once you begin dreaming with them, they can become helpful partners, pointing out the strawberries and blueberries on the table or suggesting healthy restaurants they know. And next time they invite you to their home they will ask if you have special food needs so they can be ready when you visit.

Saying No is important for success in business too. *No, I can't do that* or *I don't have time to do that* unless we shift my priorities gives your manager or leader the freedom to find someone else who can do it and will, avoiding missed deadlines, upset customers and costly disappointments. There's nothing worse than having someone say yes and not follow through, leaving you and others in the lurch.

Low self-confidence makes it hard for you to say No to others, and it makes it hard for you to say No to yourself. No to your momentary desire for that pastry on the table or the candy bar you catch sight of as you rush to your next event. No to your red-blinking-desire to abandon your food plan and go back to being heavy. To wearing the comfy fat-clothes in your closet.

You have a Success File and you also have a Failure File

Now that you know more about Success, it's time to take a closer look at failure... what it is and what it isn't.

Good news... failure is simply incompletion

Failure is <u>not</u> something to feel mad, sad or guilty about. It's <u>not</u> a reason to give up on what you want! *A failure is simply an incompletion.* An incompletion you can *now re-decide* whether you actually want to complete or delete. An incompletion that can become the seed for far more fruitful future successes.

Let's look at what is in your Failure File? And who put it there? Your mother or father? A teacher, coach or advisor? A friend or neighbor? Maybe the action or comment they made seemed insignificant *to them* at the time. Maybe they don't even remember making it now. But for you, it was stinging, painful. And most of all *unconsciously unforgettable,"* added Susan.

32

> "Until you make the unconscious conscious,
> it will direct your life and you will call it fate."
> Carl Jung

Here's one that really hurt... I failed at handwriting

Here's a childhood failure that was definitely stinging. At home I was a good little boy, polite and well-behaved. I did what I was told to do and I usually did it well. My parents were pleased and so was I. But at school I was the worst student in my class. I was well-behaved of course but, try as I might, I couldn't do what my teachers wanted me to do, the way they wanted me to do it. My handwriting was illegible. I simply couldn't form the letters.

I was scared whenever I was asked to read my homework assignment out loud to the class. I stammered and turned red because I couldn't make out my own handwriting, literally. The other kids snickered and made fun of me.

When we had exams, my classmates wrote theirs, but I had to take mine orally. Despite working with a therapist, my handwriting has failed to improve even to this day. Thank heavens for computers and cell phones, emails and texts!

What did that *old failure* force you to get good at?

"Celso, let's stop now and look a little deeper. The truth is, even in childhood, you were *never willing or able to do everything you were told, the way you were told to do it*. If you think back a little harder, you will probably discover that your *failures in others' eyes led to successes in your eyes later on.* To the development of unique parts of you! Let's look at that old failure differently this time. What else did your poor handwriting force you to become good at?" asked Susan.

Ah yes, I learned to *memorize* my homework assignments instead of trying to read them out loud. There were far fewer insults and snickers after that.

As Susan kept asking questions, I remembered two other successes my handwriting failure led me to create. As bad as I was at handwriting, that's how good I became at video games. I loved playing them. They were something I spent hours doing. In fact, I won the first Atari championship ever held in Brazil. I competed against thousands of kids and adults, and I won! That wasn't the only success which came out of that early failure either.

By the time I entered rabbinical school, I could stand and speak comfortably for hours while others in my class found memorizing sermons impossible. I could literally feel their stress and anxiety as they tried to speak... like me with my handwriting. And here's something else. As I tell you this story, it makes me laugh to think that my elementary teachers probably still believe that I ended up as a failure. In fact I connected on Facebook with one of them and she was shocked to learn that I had written a book, and even more surprised to hear that it had become a bestseller.

My success and "the success my father had in mind for me" didn't match

When I was a teenager, I told my father I wanted to buy a farm in the swampland of Brazil so I could raise alligators. Dad managed to remain calm and wisely suggested that I go to college first to learn more about alligators. Somewhere along that path, I changed my mind. Instead of raising alligators, I decided to become a Rabbi. There must be similarities that I didn't see at the time!

"Celso, even though you may no longer want to own an alligator farm there may still be some disappointment attached to that memory because you couldn't complete it at the time. To release that energy and make it available for re-use, you need to re-label that experience as *a deletion success* and let it go!" said Susan.

My father owned a company that had the third largest door-to-door catalog in South America with more than 150,000 salespeople. They made everything from cosmetics to costume jewelry, from long Mormon underwear to sexy lingerie. No doubt, what my Dad had in mind for me was taking over his business. And for several years when he was ill, I stepped in and ran the business well.

Success in my father's mind was manufacturing and selling products people wanted for a profit, but that would have been a boring life for me. I wanted to travel the world and meet lots of new people. To each his own but my Dad's own was not mine.

You don't love fish. If you loved it you would not have killed it and cooked it on a fire

As a young adult in Brazil, I heard about a program which offered to pay talented kids in the community to study Torah in the evening, Wow, I thought, I can use that money for gas or to go to the movies. They paid me $100 a month which was a huge amount of money for a young man in Brazil. And I studied in this program for several years.

Little did the program directors know that "the talkative, persuasive boy I was" came from a long line of European rabbis and my brother was already in rabbinical college.

My father's uncle developed a system of studying Talmud that is still in wide use today... read a page a day for 7 years and you will have read the whole Talmud.

My grandmother's grandfather, The Kotzker Rebbe, created sayings still relevant today like...[2]

"Where is God? Wherever you let him in."

"You don't love fish. If you loved it you would not have killed it and cooked it on a fire."

In the mid-1800s my grandmother's grandfather was the first rabbi to develop a system for training Jewish leaders. And somehow all this inherited knowledge seemed to be stored in my mind and body.

Because of my inability to write that developed into my ability to speak and discuss, I probably seemed more informed than I was, but nevertheless, I was chosen to go to America and received a full scholarship to attend rabbinical college in my mid-20s.

All the head rabbis were impressed by my persuasive abilities and I was the top scholar in one of the Kabbalah texts. Instead of getting stuck on one side of the argument or the other, I could discuss the logic of all sides and people.

Not becoming an industrialist in Brazil and not fulfilling my boyhood teacher's expectations, which looked like failures at the time, have led me to the best parts of my life. I am sure I would have been deeply depressed if I had not *failed then* and pursued my own path ever since.

What's in your Failure File?

"We all have memories that interfere with our current dreams. Old voices that tell us *you can't* or *you shouldn't*. Old scenes that make us feel we just aren't good at that, even if we haven't tried to do it for years. Old diets we started but abandoned.

What old memories could come up to haunt you? To make you feel you can't gain health or lose weight? What's in your Failure File, what incompletions are still there and when did those incompletions occur? What weren't you able to complete or delete?

What old experiences still haunt you? What were you not able to do then? What embarrassments still come to mind, and into your body when you think about them?

And who's in your Failure File?

Who's in your Failure File, whose worries and concerns may have prevented you from doing things you really wanted to do? Whose leadership let you down?

How can you now re-tell those stories, taking responsibility for not just their part but yours? Be sure to remember all the things you did that other people didn't want to you do so you can be clear, that no matter what they said or did then, you have a choice now," added Susan.

Failure Filing: Key Questions

What diets have you been on? How much weight did you lose? How much did you regain?

Whose voices talk you out of what you want to do or be? What do they say? What happened in your past that still haunts you or makes you doubt yourself?

What can you learn from past failures? What tripped you up? What old habit or way of thinking has blocked you?

Whose dreams or outcomes did you fail to complete? Your father's, mother's, teacher's or coach's? Who else's? Or was your incomplete outcome one you created? When did you create it? Do you still want it now?

Did anyone say anything about your weight that made you feel self-conscious? Were you chosen for sports teams, parties or special events? Or were you left out?

What positions or opportunities did you *fail to pursue* because of your weight? As you look back now, what did you miss out on?

What have you stopped doing because you are heavy? Bathing suits, swimming pools, dressing up, buying new clothes? Have you stopped looking for a mate or friend, a job or new home?

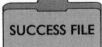

SUCCESS FILE

* Success is completion * Success is deletion *Success is creation

To jumpstart your thinking, here are some items you may be able to add to your Success File too...
bought more fruits and vegetables
paid attention to nutrients in foods I bought in grocery stores and restaurants
 read nutrition labels.
inventoried kitchen and donated food I don't want to eat
substituted whole wheat instead of white flour (*we'll discuss grain/gluten questions in detail later on)
broiled chicken breasts and fish fillets and veggies at home
began watching my sodium intake
stopped eating in restaurants where food is highly processed
cut diet soda intake from a can a day to a can a week
made soup with chicken and lots of vegetables... delicious!
made an appointment with my doctor to assess my fitness level
tried on my workout clothes in front of the mirror
started running 1 minute, walking 1 minute, then went to 2
called a gym and an exercise class to get schedule and costs
carried healthy snacks and water bottle with me

And remember to add as many past successes as you can. What successes have you had in school, in your career and family?

When your Success File is full, you feel Success-Full and self-confident. When it is low, you feel scared and unsure, dependent and needy. And needing food too!

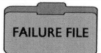

FAILURE FILE

* Failure is incompletion * Do you want to complete, delete or recreate this outcome?

List 5 Failures... 5 incompletions you or someone close to you labeled as Failures. Take some time to review each one.

When did this happen? How long ago? Was the person involved a parent, teacher, boss or spouse? Or was it you? Do old feelings (energies) still come up when you remember that experience?

Think about Celso's poor handwriting and being made fun of in school. Was your Failure in school, or was it in sports or a job? With a friend or a romance? With your weight or your health?

Look at each Failure through today's eyes and experience levels. Imagine taking a seat in the audience and observing what is happening to her or him up on a big screen like at a movie.

What can you see differently now? Were you unable to say No? Or was your No not heard? What would you do differently or ask others to do differently now? Who would you ask for help?

Like Celso, what did that failure teach you? What did it force you to get good at? How did it make you more sensitive... as a parent, a teacher, a worker or boss? As a person?

How did it change the direction of your life, from raising alligators to becoming a rabbi, a loving parent, social worker? What else?

List incompletions in your Failure File so you can update them and <u>recycle</u> that old energy to create what you want <u>now</u>.

Diet Skill Two: Updating... will your past suck you back? Or will your future pull you ahead?

The Second Success Skill is Updating. HSPs regularly update their ideas about the future, whether that updated future was living on an alligator farm or becoming a rabbi or husband or father or writer.

HSPs also update their ideas about the past. They stop to look at old situations with new eyes, today's eyes and today's experience levels. *What happened not as I saw it then, but as I am able to see it now?* How would I act and feel differently now that I have experienced life from far more perspectives? And how do I want to experience it in the future... as something I learned from or something I let hold me back?

Success skills are like tools in a toolbox

For those of you who have read other books by Susan, *The Joy of Success, Our Children Are Watching, and Shifting Gears*, you will probably notice the success skills are numbered differently in *The Miracle Diet*. Success skills are like tools in a toolbox... pliers, screwdrivers, hammers, chisels, wrenches, etc. There is no particular order in which you need to use them. So in this book, the Success Skills are numbered in the order that I used them.

Here's the bottom line... *use 'em when you need 'em!*

My father had a heart attack at 40. And so will I... or so my doctor believed

I remember hearing my doctor tell me I was genetically predisposed to having a heart attack, diabetes and high blood pressure. He said I could try diet and exercise, but he would prescribe a cholesterol-lowering medicine anyway, giving me a clear indication that he didn't think I would follow through or that, even if I did, it wouldn't help. I would still have a heart attack just like my Dad.

When my doctor handed me the prescription, he told me I would have to be on that med the rest of my life. Yes, the rest of my life! And he said I needed to have my liver checked every few months. It wasn't just my heart that was at threat. Now my liver could be damaged by the medicine as well. I was scared and hopeless. But I wasn't alone.

1 in 7 Americans takes cholesterol-lowering medicines

An estimated 1 in 7 Americans has high blood cholesterol resulting in 800,000 deaths each year. Approximately 30 million Americans take cholesterol-lowering medication, making them the most prescribed medication in the U.S. Although they help a lot of people, as with any medication, there are risks to taking these drugs. You should try to find other ways of lowering your cholesterol that might be a better option for you and your health. If those other strategies are successful, you might not need these drugs or you might be able to take a lower dose.

The key to lower cholesterol and reduced risk of heart disease is through lifestyle changes. Lifestyle changes include exercising at least 30 minutes a day on most days of the week; eating a healthy diet low in fat, cholesterol, and salt; managing stress; and quitting smoking. Even if you decide to take cholesterol-lowering medication or have been taking it for a while, these lifestyle behaviors are important for managing cholesterol. [3]

When diet and exercise fail. No, when we fail to diet and exercise

We hear over and over on TV, "When diet and exercise fail…" No, it's not when diet and exercise fail, it's when we fail to diet and exercise.

Like everyone else, I hoped there was a "magic bullet" just around the corner, but I soon realized there wasn't. I visited a congregant who had bariatric surgery with disastrous results. She used up her insurance benefits, spent several million dollars and still almost died. Sad to say, months later I performed a funeral for a congregant who chose to have his stomach stapled and months later committed suicide.

Weight and accountability… medical short cuts and bariatric surgery

A report in *The American Journal of Medicine* indicates that "patients who have bariatric surgery to lose weight have an increased risk of suicide compared with the general population. But the reasons for the pattern, researchers say, remain unknown."[4]

Fortunately tragedies like these can be avoided when we knowingly say YES and NO to foods that are offered to us.

Liposuction… fat can come back in lumps and bumps

When Oprah's infamous rapid weight loss liquid diet was the craze, Dr. Pamela Peak met a woman she'll never forget. "She'd dropped 90 pounds over a short period of time downing 600 calories a day of some pricey fluid concoction. Here's the catch. She'd done it three times for a total of 270 pounds worth of yo-yo'ing. During that time, she'd endured extensive liposuction and skin tightening procedures... When she opened her patient gown, I was saddened to see railroad tracks of stretched scarring, which I had expected. What was unusual were her fat deposits. She felt like a freak, with lumps and bumps pouching out around her overstretched scars. It just broke my heart."

Dr. Peak continued to see the same lumps and bumps in other patients who regained weight after liposuction. "In fact, it was so common that I warned people ahead of time — *If you want to do liposuction, don't regain the weight.*"

Liposuction can remove up to two to three pounds of fat below the skin. But the fat deep inside the abdomen and around the organs is the fat that really matters. This toxic fat is associated with heart disease and diabetes and can never be lipo'd. "The only way to reduce that fat load to normal levels is through healthy lifestyle choices."[5]

Whether it's bariatric surgery or liposuction, you need to permanently change your lifestyle to get the results you want.

I knew my Creator didn't mean for me to be fat, sick or lumpy

I had to update what my doctor had told me. I was confident I could heal myself if I was willing to work with God. And I have. Since losing 100 pounds and exercising 6 days a week for more than a year, my cholesterol has been a perfect 114. My triglycerides are 1/3 of what they used to be. And my blood sugar is 'athletically' low.

Be careful who you listen to! Even a well-intentioned doctor can plant a powerful negative outcome in your mind, an outcome that scares you instead of empowers you to change your diet and exercise, to change your health and life. I knew my Creator didn't mean for me to be fat, sick or lumpy. Otherwise he would have made me that way.

You are what you eat, but what are you eating?

We have all heard people say *you are what you eat,* and yes, it is true. God's foods make us feel healthy and energetic but when we experience blood sugar highs and lows, when our brain is not receiving the nutrients it needs, our confidence is thrown off. We must nourish ourselves properly so we can feel confident and energetic, *from the inside out.*

The Honey story… a lesson taught by a dog
It's not what we want to eat but what our bodies need

Here's something Susan learned from her dog. "My gentle dog Honey who met Celso at the door the first time he came to my home is a fine example of what a change in diet can do for you. It isn't always a question of mind over matter, sometimes it's a question of matter over mind. Or how well we are nourishing our body despite what the experts say. Take Honey for example, she loved the kibble I was feeding her and she loved to pick up wrappers with tiny bits of leftover hamburgers and fries she found along the street when we went out for walks, but eating what Honey liked simply wasn't working for her body.

I was feeding Honey the best grain-free, dry dog food on the market and giving her the best flea prevention meds… according to the experts I consulted, but Honey was constantly itching and scratching, especially at night when I was trying to sleep. Honey was chewing bald spots in her coat and her hair was falling out.

I went to the internet and searched for "no fleas but dog scratches and chews" and several articles came up suggesting I take Honey off processed, dry food and put her on fresh chicken and vegetables. So I decided to try it. I bought organic chicken thighs, bags of broccoli and carrots, poured them in a large pot and brought them just to a boil. This healthy dog soup lasts for two days.

Within three weeks, Honey's shiny new fur was already growing in and I was getting sleep. And everyone who walks early mornings with me says Honey is much slimmer and looks like a new dog. She runs like the wind in joyous, giant circles in the grassy field. If it could happen for Honey, it can happen for you! From processed to home cooked, it made a big difference."

A diet is a marathon, not a sprint

The first thought most people have about diets is, I'll do this for a couple of weeks or months. Then I'll go back to my old, enjoyable ways. *No, going back to your old ways simply won't work.* A diet is a marathon, not a sprint! The sooner you realize it, the sooner you will be able to permanently change your weight and your health.

Fat cells have memories. They want to go back to their old size. But new muscles have memories too and, once you have created muscles, they work hard to hold your new shape.

You are always on a diet. The only question is, a diet for what? Health or obesity? Longevity or illness?

My before pictures are now a source of joy

My before pictures which used to embarrass me are one of my most prized possessions today. A source of joy... one of the most satisfying and profound accomplishments I have had in my life.

At 35, I looked 50. At 40, I looked 40.

But now at 42, after *The Miracle Diet*, people say I look like I'm in my 30s. But I feel better than I did in my 20s… stronger, more flexible and more energetic. Without any surgery.

The only thing operating on me was my God-given renewing body and his miraculous healing foods.

Remember, you must change your mind to change your weight

"You can have all the right foods in your refrigerator or on your restaurant menu and still not eat them. *You've got to change your mind to change your weight and your health!*

Voices from your past will haunt you until you update them

Lingering feelings of failure indicate that you need to re-imagine that past experience. Old energy, new energy… energy is energy. Once you release it, it will become available to re-use in desirable new ways. In ways that will fulfill not just yesterday's but today's and tomorrow's dreams.

You may have been stuck in one-and-only-one point of view… *your view at the time*. But how long ago was that? What have you learned since? Take charge now. Be the director of that old scene, rechoose your cast, move "your mental camera" and retake the scene the way you would want it to do now. Experience the details of that version so your brain can start searching for opportunities to actually live and enjoy it. Opportunities to experience the kind of support you want, the kind of communication and encouragement. The success.

Be sure to think in detail about *what you would want instead*. Create those positive success experiences and take a few minutes to imagine stepping in and experiencing them," urged Susan.

Updating what you know about food and how it works in your body

Unfortunately today we are no longer eating the foods God designed to renew our bodies. We have started de-constructing and re-engineering His foods, adding chemicals so they can last longer on store shelves. We are over-planting, over-fertilizing, over-spraying and depleting our soil. And we have failed to notice the profound cost... the loss of vital, essential nutrients God has in mind for us. The loss of our health.

Instead of hunting and gathering, instead of farming and harvesting in the area where we live, we are flying God's fruits and vegetables around the planet, not eating foods designed for our terrain and climate. We are distributing, selling and consuming "fresh foods" (or so the package says) days and weeks after they have been harvested.

Have you heard the buzz about the bees?

Even the bees God provided to pollinate our crops and fruit trees are moved around the country instead of living where they were born and bees are mysteriously disappearing with potentially disastrous consequences. Without something as tiny as a bee, the nurturing, nourishing world God created for us could come undone. And the bodies God created for us could come undone too. It's up to us now.

We have abundance but we also have limiting habits. We have narrowed our choices to just a few foods... the ones we regularly pick up in the aisles of our favorite stores. Certain brands and sizes. And we buy the same few every week. We have come to think of fruits, vegetables, fish and animals as packaged products in cardboard, metal and plastic, instead of life-renewing nutrients for our self-healing bodies.

There's more to salt than salt

The discovery that salt could preserve food was a powerful leap forward for early man. Salt-preserved foods meant they were no longer dependent on the seasonal availability of foods and so they could travel greater distances. Salt was hard to come by and highly prized in trade. Even the likes of Marco Polo were in pursuit of salt.

Travels of Marco Polo in the 1200s

Here are Marco Polo's own words from *The Travels of Marco Polo*, Book 1 Chapter 28:

"After those twelve days' journey you come to a fortified place called Taican. It is a fine place, and the mountains that you see towards the south are all composed of salt. People from all the countries round, to some thirty days' journey, come to fetch this salt, which is the best in the world, and is so hard that it can only be broken with iron picks. 'Tis in such abundance that it would supply the whole world to the end of time."[6] Note: Now Taican is in Afghanistan.

But if Marco Polo could see how much salt we use today, he would no doubt retract his statement.

We are fed by profit-oriented manufacturers

Instead of fed by God, we are fed by profit-making manufacturers who reduce fresh whole foods to highly sugared, highly salted addictive products. To high calorie, fiber-less, high-sugar juices instead of whole fruits and vegetables. To fried foods instead of fresh, quickly sautéed or steamed ones. To fast foods in huge portions with huge quantities of salt, sugar and fat.

How does salt preserve food?

Salt preserves food in two ways. One, like mummification, salt removes water from cells, effectively drying them out. Two, salt kills some of the bacteria and fungi that cause food to spoil by removing water from them as well.

Salt versus Sodium

Though the terms are often used interchangeably, salt and sodium are *not* the same. Table salt (sodium chloride NaCl) is composed of 40% sodium and 60% chloride. Sodium is the part of salt you need to be aware of.

How much sodium is in a teaspoon of salt?

One teaspoon of salt contains 2,360 mg of sodium. We add salt during cooking and at the table. Manufacturers add it too, and frequently in great quantities, to help preserve processed foods and restore flavor they lost during processing. When you read nutrition content labels, you need to look for *sodium*.

Daily sodium recommendations

The USDA Dietary Guidelines for Americans (2010) recommends that adult men and women consume less than 2,300 mg of sodium per day, and 1,500 mg or less if you are over 50 or African American, have high blood pressure, diabetes or chronic kidney disease.[7] However, the American Heart Association recommends that *everyone* should consume less than 1,500 mg of sodium per day.[8] That means that one teaspoon of salt, (which contains approximately 2,400 mg of sodium) far exceeds that recommendation.

But on average, Americans consume far more sodium than that. American men eat between 3,100 and 4,700 mg of sodium per day. American women eat between 2,300 to 3,100 mg because they usually have a lower calorie intake.

"The importance of the association between excess salt intake and raised blood pressure— leading, in turn, to strokes and coronary heart disease—cannot be overstated," says Dr. Lawrence J. Appel, a professor of medicine at the Johns Hopkins University School of Medicine.[9]

Blood pressure is the force of blood pushing against blood vessel walls. When you eat too much salt, which contains 40% sodium, your body holds extra water to "wash" the salt from your body. In some people, this may cause blood pressure to rise, putting stress on your heart and blood vessels.

Salt and water balance... God's original design

Why is sodium intake so important? Sodium is an electrolyte which facilitates electrical signaling in the body, allowing muscles to fire and the brain to work. For our bodies to function properly, the concentration of electrolytes must stay balanced.

Here's how sodium balancing and rebalancing works. This is especially important when you increase your exercise or exercise where it's hot. A high concentration of electrolytes triggers thirst. When we drink enough water, our kidneys maintain that concentration by increasing or decreasing the amount of water we retain.

When we eat more salt, water moves from our bloodstream into our skin, giving us that "puffy" look and making it hard to pull off our rings. When we eat less salt, the process works in reverse removing excess water from our bodies.

Hydration, hydration, hydration... drink more, but how much?

Water makes up about 60 percent of your weight. How much water should you drink to keep that up level? Easy to ask, but not so easy to answer. Like so many other things in life, it depends.

Do you live in a temperate climate, a tropical one or a desert? Do you exercise a lot or a little? Do you work outside or inside? Do you eat a lot of juicy fruits and vegetables? Do you carry a water bottle and drink throughout the day, or just when you're thirsty?

The Institute of Medicine says men need about 13 cups or 3 liters of total beverages a day. And women need about 9 cups or 2.2 liters a day. Lack of water can lead to dehydration, a condition that comes from not having enough water in your body to carry out normal functions. Even mild dehydration can drain your energy and make you feel tired.

Dehydration occurs when fluid loss exceeds fluid intake. We lose water every day in our breath, sweat, urine and stool. Along with water, we also lose small amounts of electrolytes including salt.

Signs of dehydration include increased thirst, dry mouth, weakness or lightheadedness (particularly if worse on standing), darkening of or decrease in urination. Severe dehydration can lead to changes in the body chemistry, kidney failure, and death.

Vitamin C can make a life and death difference

Scurvy was common among sailors, pirates and passengers on voyages at sea that lasted longer than perishable fruits and vegetables could be stored. They survived on cured and salted meats and dried grains.

During months at sea, early American colonists died in droves before ever reaching land. Some shiploads arrived half full... until ship owners made sure travel routes took them to tropical islands along the way where they could get citrus to ensure their survival. Where they could get vitamin C to prevent scurvy.

Salt has no calories but salty foods do

You might be surprised to learn that salt has no calories but is frequently associated with weight gain. High levels of salt in our diet *do not come from fresh foods from the garden* but from calorie-packed, fiber-deficient, processed-foods found in fast foods, restaurants and on supermarket shelves. Sodium intake is one factor in the development of high blood pressure or hypertension which tends to develop as we age.

Here's something important to keep in mind as you raise children. There are indications that high sodium intake early in life may weaken one's genetic defenses against developing high blood pressure later on. Can you imagine what this means for our future? Experts recommend reducing sodium while your blood pressure is still normal. So start teaching your children which foods to eat and which ones to avoid because they contain excessive salt.

"The importance of cutting down on salt to reduce dietary sodium hasn't really hit home with many consumers either, experts say. And the food industry has resisted tougher regulations on salt content, even though more than 70% of the salt in the U.S. diet comes from packaged foods, not the salt shaker,"proclaims *The Tufts University Health & Nutrition Letter*, March 1, 2010.

How much additional sodium do you add as you cook and at the table? How much do restaurants add... and why?

To the left in the following chart, you can see the sodium content of the food as God created it. Moving to the right, you see how much extra sodium is added to that food as it is processed and prepared, from apple to apple pie, from tomato to tomato sauce, from cucumber to dill pickle, from pork to ham.

Sodium comparisons: God's foods versus manufacturers' foods			
Little	**Low**	**More**	**High**
Apple, 1--2 mg	**Applesauce**, 1 c.--6 mg	**Apple pie**, 1/8, frozen--208 mg	**Apple pie**, 1, fast food--400 mg
Low sodium bread, 1 slice--7 mg	**Bread**, 1 slice, white--114 mg	**Pound cake**, 1 slice--171 mg	**English muffin**, 1 whole--203 mg
Vegetable oil, 1 tbsp.--0 mg	**Butter**, 1 tbsp., unsalted--2 mg	**Butter**, 1 tbsp., salted--116	**Margarine**, 1 tbsp.--140 mg
Chicken, 1/2 breast--69 mg	**Chicken pot pie**, 1, frozen--907 mg	**Chicken noodle soup,** 1 c.--1,107 mg	**Chicken dinner**, fast food--2,243 mg
Fresh corn, 1 ear--1 mg	**Frozen corn**, 1 c.--7 mg	**Corn flakes**, 1 c.--256 mg	**Canned corn**, 1 c.--384 mg
Cucumber, 7 slices--2 mg	**Sweet pickle**, 1--128 mg	**Cucumber w/salad dressing**--234 mg	**Dill pickle**, 1,928 mg
Pork, 3 oz.--59 mg	**Bacon**, 4 slices--548 mg	**Frankfurter**, 1--639 mg	**Ham**, 3 oz.--1,114 mg
Lemon, 1--1 mg	**Catsup**, 1 tbsp.--	**Soy sauce**, 1 tbsp.--	**Salt,** 1 tsp.--1,938

	156 mg	1,029 mg	mg
Potato, 1--5 mg	**Potato chips**, 10--200 mg	**Mashed potatoes**, instant, 1 c.--485 mg	**Potato salad**, 1/2 cup--625 mg
Plain yogurt, 1 c.--105 mg	**Milk**, 1 c.--122 mg	**Buttermilk**, 1 c.--257 mg	**Choc. pudding**, 1/2 c. instant--470 mg
Steak, 3 oz.--55 mg	**Corned beef**, 3 oz.--802 mg	**Jumbo burger**, fast food--990 mg	**Meat loaf**, frozen dinner--1,304 mg
Tomato, 1--14 mg	**Tomato juice**, 1 c.--878 mg	**Tomato soup**, 1 c.--932 mg	**Tomato sauce**, 1 c.--1,498 mg
Tuna, fresh, 3 oz.--50 mg	**Tuna**, canned, 3 oz.--384 mg	**Tuna pot pie**, 1 frozen--715 mg	**Fish sandwich**, 1, fast food--882 mg
Peanuts, unsalted, 1 c.--8 mg	**Peanut butter**, 1 tbsp.--81 mg	**Peanut brittle**, 1 oz.--145 mg	**Dry roasted peanuts**, salted, 1 c.--986 mg
Low sodium cheddar, 1 oz.--6 mg	**Cheddar cheese**, 1 oz.--176 mg	**Cottage cheese**, 1/2 cup--257 mg	**American cheese**, 1 oz.--406 mg
Water, 8 oz., tap--12 mg	**Club soda**, 8 oz.--39 mg	**Antacid in water**--564 mg	**Beef bouillon**, 8 oz.--1,152 mg

Keep this number in mind as you study this chart.

1 tsp. salt = approximately 2,400 mg[10]

What happens when we cook at home instead of eating out?

When you broil or grill a 6 oz skinless chicken breast and you do not add oil, butter or salt that piece of chicken has 192 calories or less (some of the fat drips off and is poured away) and 128 mg of sodium. But if you buy it at Kentucky Fried Chicken, that 6 oz of chicken breast has 400 calories and 1145 mg sodium. But how many people, especially teens, *only* eat 6 oz of Kentucky Fried chicken?

If you broil 6 oz of 95% lean ground beef that burger will have 295 calories or less and 120 mg sodium. But if you eat a Big MAC that burger will contain 540 calories and 1040 mg sodium. A Whopper has even more calories... 733 calories and 1000 mg sodium! And most people simply say they ate a burger.

Why do American food manufacturers use grams instead of ounces in Nutrition Lists on products?

Which is it grams or ounces? The use of grams is bit confusing for those of us who didn't grow up thinking metric and are used to buying our food in ounces.[11] Do you know how to convert grams into ounces? No? I didn't either. So here it is just in case you are mathematically inclined.

1 Ounce = 28.3495231 Grams

Grill This, Not That!

In their book, *Grill This, Not That!,* Zinczenko and Goulding say, "Red Lobster's Cedar Plank Salmon might sound like a safe bet, but it actually has 1,050 calories and 40g of fat, 9 grams of which are the artery-clogging saturated kind. Restaurants keep marinating with butter and fat whereas on your home grill the fat burns off. Besides you can decide whether and what to marinade your food with... herbs, salt and pepper, brown sugar? You'll know what has been added and avoid thousands of hidden calories and *as much as 3 days worth of sodium.*"[12]

Just so you know, before it is cooked...
6 oz fresh Wild Atlantic Salmon has 241 calories
6 oz fresh Farm Raised Atlantic Salmon has 330 calories.

Here's something else you should know... chicken skin has 100 calories

Most of us remember sneaking in the kitchen as kids and pulling crispy, golden skin off our Mom' hot roast chicken or turkey. And getting yelled at for ruining her meal. Yes, chicken skin is delicious, but eater beware. Here are the facts.

On average, a 6 oz. piece of white meat chicken breast with skin has approximately 340 calories. If you remove the skin, it will have about 165 calories... less than half the calories. Chicken skin contains an alarming amount of fat. A 6 oz skinless piece of chicken breast contains a mere 3 g of fat, but that same piece of chicken with skin on it contains a whopping 14 g of fat.

Your backyard garden offers the best produce

Fresh foods are best and fresh foods from your garden are the best of the best. Crispy green peas right off the vine. Red juicy tomatoes still warm from the sun. Carrots with earth hanging from tiny rootlets and lacy green tops still attached. Freezing, drying, cooking and reheating reduce nutrients. Nearly all food preparation steps lower the nutrients in food, especially when it is exposed to high levels of heat, light or oxygen.

Nutrients can also be "washed out." When you boil a potato many B and C vitamins go into the water. You can still benefit from those nutrients if you drink the liquid or add it to soups, but not if you pour it down the drain. Similar losses happen when you broil, roast or fry food in oil and drain off the drippings.

7-13 cups of produce daily

The U.S. government's dietary guidelines suggest we eat *7-13 cups* of produce daily. Make sure you stock your kitchen with plenty of fresh fruits and vegetables and have a few servings at each meal to boost your intake of healthful vitamins, minerals, antioxidants, phytochemicals and fiber. Remember, if you fill up on low-calorie, nutrient-dense fruits and vegetables, you'll be less likely to binge on highly-processed snacks and juices.

How many calories do manufacturers add?

Check out these comparisons...

1 whole orange (1 c) 84.6 calories
1 c orange juice 112 calories. A 32% increase.

1 c fresh pineapple 83 calories
1 c unsweetened pineapple juice 133 calories. A 37.5% increase.

And the fiber has been removed too.

Fiber is a carbohydrate the body doesn't break down so it doesn't add any calories. In fact, according to the Joslin Diabetes Center, an affiliate of the Harvard Medical School, the grams of fiber can be subtracted from the total grams of carbohydrate if you are using carb counting for meal planning.[13]

Not only does food processing... juicing, bottling, canning and distributing... cost a lot of time and money but it also removes valuable calorie-subtracting fiber, reduces freshness, nutrients and usually adds sugar.

Besides water, what do you drink?

Coffee or tea? Do you add milk, cream or sugar? Or do you let Starbucks, Dunkin Donuts or McDonalds add it for you? Coffee has next to no calories. A cup of black coffee contains only about 1 calorie from small traces of oil in coffee beans.

You can get your coffee in any of Starbuck's sizes, Tall, Grande and Venti, and they all still have less than 3 calories *unless* you opt to buy one of their far more enticing delicacies. A Light Frappuccino Grande has 140 calories and I occasionally enjoy one after a long walk.

Don't kid yourself into believing "Starbucks milkshakes" are "coffees"

No or low calorie coffee, no. Their White Hot Chocolate whip is far richer at 1070 calories. And that tasty little chocolate peanut butter bar you purchase as an add-on has 730 calories. So 1070 plus 730 equals more than the number of calories you will probably want to eat in a day.[9]

Here's something new... Very Berry Hibiscus Starbucks Refreshers

Fruit juice and whole blackberries shaken with Green Coffee Extract for a boost of natural energy, served over ice. 70 calories. A low-calorie afternoon recharge that tastes nothing like coffee.

If you regularly eat in specific restaurants, ask them how they prepare your food. Added fat? Salt? Sugar? Calories?

Sugar and cheaper high fructose corn syrup

Here in South Florida, we can still see sugar cane growing and we buy cane juice fresh squeezed. Delicious but not too sweet. Sugar is a 6-19 foot tall grass that waves in our warm breezes. Its stem or cane is the source of 80% of the sugar we consume. Most of the rest comes from sugar beets. Sugarcane is the world's largest crop. Yes, that's right, the world's largest crop. Sadly sugar cane severely depletes the soil and in Brazil there are areas that are becoming deserts as a result.

In 1977 sugar quotas on imported sugar increased the cost significantly so U.S. producers found cheaper sources. High-fructose corn syrup is economical because the price of corn is kept artificially low by government subsidies paid to growers. Soft drink makers such as Coca-Cola and Pepsi still use *sugar in other nations,* but they switched to high-fructose corn syrup in the U.S. in 1984.[14]

Do you recognize all these names of sugars?

Always read the ingredients list. Foods you might not even realize are sweetened, like bread, dried fruits and crackers, might be hiding added sugars. Learn to identify terms that mean sugar, including white sugar, brown sugar, cane sugar, confectioner's sugar, corn syrup, crystallized fructose, dextrin, dextran, dextrose, diastatic malt, diatase, d-mannose, honey, invert sugar, maple syrup, raw sugar, beet sugar, cane sugar, corn sweeteners, evaporated cane juice, glucose-fructose, granulated fructose, high fructose corn syrup, fructose, malt, maltose, molasses, and turbinado sugar. Try to limit foods that have any of these "sugars" *as one of the first three ingredients*, keeping in mind that ingredients are listed in order of highest to lesser content. Easy to make us think we are eating less sugar, isn't it?

Glycemic Index

The glycemic index (GI) is a measure of the effect of carbohydrates consumed on blood sugar. The higher the number, the greater the blood sugar response. So a low GI food will cause a small rise, while a high GI food will trigger a dramatic spike. By definition, glucose has a GI of 100. Other foods have a lower GI.

Classification	GI range	Examples
Low GI	55 or less	most fruits and vegetables; legumes/pulses; some whole, intact grains; nuts; tagatose; fructose; kidney beans; beets; chickpeas
Medium GI	56–69	whole wheat products, basmati rice, sweet potato, sucrose (table sugar), baked potatoes
High GI	70 and above	white bread, most white rices, corn flakes, *extruded breakfast cereals*, glucose, maltose, maltodextrins (sugars)

*Extruded breakfast cereals

An extruder is an industrial machine that produces little flakes, O's and puffed up grains using high temperatures and pressures. The cereal industry has convinced the FDA that extruded grains are no different from non-extruded grains and seem to have managed to block the publishing of studies of their effects on humans and animals. However, two unpublished animal studies indicate that extruded grains are toxic, particularly to the nervous system. Further testing is needed.

The glycemic load (GL) is a newer way to understand the effect of carbohydrates in foods that gives a fuller picture. A GI value tells you *how rapidly* a particular carbohydrate turns into sugar, but it doesn't tell you *how much* carbohydrate is in a serving of that food. You need to know both to understand that food's effect on blood sugar. For example, the carbohydrate in watermelon has a high GI but there isn't a lot of carbohydrate in it, so watermelon's GL is relatively low. A GL of 20 or more is high, a GL of 11 to 19 is medium, and a GL of 10 or less is low.[15]

More shocking Glycemic Index facts... whole grain bread raises blood sugar more than some candy bars

Dr. William Davis, a preventive cardiologist writes in his book *Wheat Belly*, "People are usually shocked when I tell them that whole wheat bread increases blood sugar to a higher level than sucrose (table sugar.) Aside from some extra fiber, eating two slices of whole wheat bread is really little different, and *often worse, than drinking a can of sugar sweetened soda or eating a sugary candy bar."*[16]

Shocking information but not new. In 1981, the original study at University of Toronto stated the GI of white bread was 69, whole wheat bread was 72, Shredded Wheat cereal was 67 and sucrose (table sugar) was 59. *Yes, the GI of whole grain bread is higher than table sugar!*

"Incidentally, the GI of a Mars bar—nougat, chocolate, sugar, caramel, and all—is 68. That's better than whole wheat grain. The GI of a Snicker's Bar is 41—*far* better than whole grain bread," adds Dr. Davis.

The GI value of Coca Cola is 63, Ocean Spray Cranberry juice cocktail 68, Gatorade 78, unsweetened Apple juice 44, unsweetened Orange juice 50 and canned Tomato juice 38.[17]

Coke or juice… is there really "a sugar difference?"

When you travel the world, the product that universally represents the U.S. is Coke. What is in Coke? You probably don't know because it's a secret… a secret, trademarked, dark brown, sweetened water.

How many teaspoons of sugar does a Coke contain? And how about fruit juice? Marshall Brain does a fascinating experiment on YouTube to discover how much sugar is in a 12 oz coke. And how much sugar is in an equal amount of fruit juice. Fun way to teach your kids.[18]

First he boils down coke to a dark sugary mass and measures it. And voila, his number matches the amount of sugar stated on the can, but the number there is given in grams (39 gm) which few of us know how to translate. 39 grams is 7 ½ teaspoons. In case you think, "Well then, I'll drink fruit juice instead." Juice contains exactly the same amount of sugar!

The real shocker is that 24 oz sodas so many kids drink these days contain 78 gm which translates to *15 teaspoons*. Yes, a huge white granular mound of sugar. And then manufacturers add 50 mg of sodium just for good measure. So instead of coke or juice, drink water!

Here's the bottom line on American fast food… a mountain of salt *and* a mountain of sugar. Marco Polo would no doubt be doubly amazed. So much food in stores and restaurants and so little nutrition left in it. But you can change that now!

The Tell-Yourself-the-Truth Inventory

Step one... Inventory what you eat and drink and what it contains

If you usually eat at home, go to your kitchen and take a close look at what's in your refrigerator, cabinets and cupboards? How much fresh food do you have on hand... salad, broccoli, asparagus, red peppers, celery, carrots, apples or bananas? Fresh or frozen meat and fish? What is usually on your shopping list? Next time you shop, be sure to read Nutrition Labels. Figure out how many calories are in *the serving sizes you consume*, not the serving sizes manufacturers recommend on the package? One sardine can we looked at says it contains 2 ½ servings!

Chances are what's in your kitchen is what you eat... including ice cream in your freezer, cookies in your cabinet, fast foods from menus on your refrigerator and restaurants on Speed Dial!

What do you snack on? Fresh fruits? Cut vegetables? Dried fruits? Cookies, cakes, ice cream? Chocolate and candy? Sweet or salty? Doritos, pretzels or potato chips? When do you overeat? Throughout the day? Before or at lunch? Before or after dinner?

Read labels! If you can't pronounce most of the ingredients, chances are the product is designed for *shelf life not your life*. What has been taken out of your food and what else has been added? Even "fresh frozen chicken" can have brine or salt added. Check sodium content. You may be quite surprised.

Step two: For the next week, keep a log of *everything* you eat or drink

Yes, everything. You need to establish a **baseline** as you begin to make changes.

What do you usually eat for breakfast... eggs, cereal, bagels or muffins? What else? How many carbs, proteins and calories do those foods contain? What do you drink or snack on during the morning, at home, in the car or at work?

What do you regularly eat for lunch? Do you eat lunch at home or bring it from home? If not, where does it come from... take outs, your cafeteria at work or restaurants? Do you know how it is prepared and what it contains? Can you find out? Do you snack in the afternoon? Fruit, nuts, food bars or candy? Exactly what do you eat or drink?

How about dinner? Do you eat at home or do you usually eat out? Where? What do you order? What portion sizes do you consume? Do you eat bread and butter? How about dessert? What do you drink besides water... alcohol, regular or diet soda or other? Do you also drink coffee or tea? Do you add sugar and cream? What else do you eat or drink before bedtime? Do you snack while watching TV, eat at bedtime or in the middle of the night? What time do you usually get to sleep and wake up? How much sleep do you get?

Remember, 1 cup of vegetables is 30-50 calories and 1 cup of brown rice or mashed potatoes is about 250 calories. You can *feel full* without consuming extra calories... more about *satiation mechanisms* in your stomach wall later on.

OK, now take a few minutes to add all this up. What is your total calorie intake per day?

Step three: Update your shopping habits... spend more time around the edges of your grocery store

This week shop strategically. Make a list. Shop when you are full, never when you are hungry! Know your store's layout. Head directly for what you want so marketers can't entice you to buy what gives them the greatest profit and you the least nutrition.

Start with fruits and vegetables. Spring mix greens and fresh spinach are a great buy. As you cook fish or chicken filets with a little olive oil in a skillet, add a large mound of greens on top in the final minutes. They reduce drastically as they cook! Steaming or microwaving green beans, kale, collards and broccoli only takes a few minutes. You can cook and mash cauliflower just like white potatoes. Sweet potatoes and yams provide added fiber and sweetness. Brussels sprouts, asparagus and eggplant are delicious broiled with a little olive oil and Kosher salt. Eat carrots fresh or steamed. You may be surprised to learn that the typical carrot has traveled 1,838 miles by the time it gets to your plate! How much petroleum has it taken to get them there? How much nutrition has they lost? Fresh from the garden, hardly? More later.

Temperate-climate fruits like apples, peaches, plums and pears tend to contain less natural sugar than tropical fruits like bananas, pineapple, mangoes and papaya. Dates contain the most sugar. Berries contain the least. Eat lots of fresh blueberries, strawberries, raspberries and blackberries. Or buy them frozen. Check labels so you can avoid brands that have added sugar and chemicals.

Eat healthy snacks. If you are overly hungry, you'll grab for anything and it probably won't be what you need... unless you brought it with you. You will have to become a food-survivalist to stay healthy and trim in today's fast food jungle. You can carry almonds in your pocket. Keep a protein bar or drink in your car, office or TV room. If you pass a convenience store you can usually find an apple or banana near the cashier.

Buy *guilt-free, all-you-can-eat snacks* like celery, carrots, cucumbers and apples. Dip in a *little* hummus, non-hydrogenated peanut or almond butter. Instead of ice cream enjoy unsweetened frozen berries and grapes. Purchase unsweetened fruit pouches designed for making smoothies and enjoy them for snacks.

How much liquid are you drinking daily? Instead of soft drinks, regular and diet, drink water, seltzer or green tea. More about these recommendations later on.

This week buy restaurant and fast food more strategically too! Ask how foods you usually eat are prepared and ask for nutritional information as well.

This is an Obesity Epidemic of our own making

Our miraculous renewing bodies are struggling to survive without the miraculous foods that God designed to fuel them. It's time to wake up and notice what we have done, and what you can do about it now! In the name of convenience, are we creating obesity and early death?

Remember, you can have all the right foods in your refrigerator or on the restaurant menu and still not eat them! You can know what you should eat and still not eat it. You've got to change your mind to change your weight and your health. *The Tell-Yourself-the-Truth Inventory is a powerful first step!*

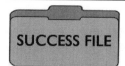

SUCCESS FILE

Diet Skill Two: Updating what you eat
and what you know about food

As you read, what did you notice about what you and your family have been eating weekdays and weekends? What are you planning to eat more and less of? To buy more and less of? What tiny thinking changes have you already made?

Review this skill and see what hit you in the head! Write down the changes you plan to make and how and when you plan to implement these changes. Yes, write your plan down!

What familiar food habits (remember, the word *familiar* come from the word *family*) have created your weight gain? The first step in change is awareness. You are already more aware!

How much wheat, sugar, fat and salt have you been consuming? Where have you been getting it? Take a good hard look at the ingredient lists of the products you regularly consume at home, in restaurants and take outs.

Food is fuel. What else do you use food for...pleasure, reward, relaxation? How else can you get these results and lose weight as well?

What excuses have you noticed yourself using? What negative thoughts have you been having? What old scenes have flashed back and caused pain? Take some time to re-live those scenes as successes this time. Direct the scene so it turns out the way you wanted it to turn out then. *Feel the feelings you wanted to feel.*

Diet Skill Three: Shifting Gears... starting, accelerating and creating your weight loss

"Here is something that HSPs do know that you probably don't. What we mean by success shifts, *and what we need to do to succeed keeps shifting too.*

Success has three gear-like phases. When you succeed, just as when you drive, you need to use *the right success gear at the right time.* If you use the wrong one, your success will jerk and stall the same way a car does when you are using the wrong gear.

Here is another reason why remembering your successes is so challenging. *Successes look and feel different in each gear so you may not have been able to recognize them.* Once you learn more in this chapter, you will be able to easily identify far more successes... 1st, 2nd and 3rd gear successes... you will be able to build your self-confidence even more.

Making your workout work for you

Ok, now that you are improving your eating and no doubt feeling better, it's time to take the next step... increasing your exercise. Heading out to walk, run, swim or workout at the gym.

What gear you will need before heading for the gym? Some would say shoes, shorts, water bottles or gloves. But no, *the most important gear you will need is the right success gear, at the right time.*

1st gear is for starting

First gear is for moving an idea, like exercising or dieting, into action. For overcoming avoidance, fear and resistance. For learning the basics of your new skill or approach. For starting to make changes in any area of your life.

Your knee is inoperable. Learn to live with it

After my orthopedic surgeon told me my knee was inoperable, "Learn to live with it," and I headed for the door, he mentioned Bikram Yoga... hot sweaty yoga. I paused as he added, "Susan, if you could do Bikram, it would strengthen your muscles and increase your flexibility." That was enough for me. I knew I was going to do it.

I remember all too well my first day at Bikram Yoga. I was definitely in 1st gear! I had never done much yoga, and even that was years ago. I couldn't' bend my left knee to 90 degrees and I certainly couldn't reach down and grab my bent knee from behind like everyone else could. So I did the best I could.

I had torn my left meniscus and a baker's cyst (a pouch of fluid) had formed behind it and grown so large that it ruptured, filling my leg with fluid and swelling it to triple. The pain was horrendous, especially at night when there was little else to distract me. I had spent hours each day lying on the couch and endured six months of painful physical therapy. So to say the least, I wasn't in good shape as I began. But I was committed to healing my knee.

After calling to find out costs and class times, I headed for my first session, slowly and uncomfortably pulling my left knee into the drivers' side of my car because it wouldn't bend on its own. Bending my knee easily and without pain was my prime goal for taking this class.

Are you and your expert in sync?

I explained my injury in detail to the teacher. I told her I needed to stand near the wall so if I lost my balance, I could fall on the wall and not on my left knee. She was hesitant and said what I was asking was a bit unorthodox. I think she expected me to say yes and comply, but I insisted that if this class was going to work for me, I would have to take care of myself first. Finally she said yes, I could stand by the wall.

Fortunately for me, I arrived at the studio at the same time that Gigi did. She was another student in the class, visibly in great shape and highly experienced. She welcomed me and told me where the bathroom was, where to put my belongings and lay down my mat. She reminded me to silence my cell phone, explained about skidless mats (they're like kids' pajamas with little plastic gripper dots on the underside) and showed me how to sprinkle water on top to make them even safer. I was afraid, deathly afraid of falling and slipping back into those months of overwhelming pain! Tentative and hesitant I was committed to my recovery. I was in 1st gear. Gigi also told me to drink plenty of water and replenish my electrolytes. I noticed that she was drinking coconut water and I chuckled to think that coconuts grow in areas where it's hot and sweaty, where electrolytes are naturally lost. Just another one of God's miraculous designs.

Standing and staring at myself in the mirror, we began. At first I had a hard time following my teacher's instructions and had to adjust some of them to respect my body. Lock your knee. Lock your knee? I couldn't even straighten it, much less lock it! It was hard for me to stare at myself in the mirror and harder still to avoid comparing myself to others in the class.

Day by day my strength and flexibility were improving. I could see it, and others in my class could see it too, generously pointing out my progress and courage, and it took a lot of courage at first. It helped that I had bought a month's pass and wanted to get my money's worth... and my health's worth of course.

A few weeks later a new student came in and started asking questions *of me*. Like Gigi, I told her where the bathroom was and where to leave her clothes, about my skidless mat and how I sprinkle water on it so I don't slip. Seeing that new student's first day showed me how far I had come. How well I could follow instructions now. How easily I could balance and stand. How much stronger I was and how much tighter my body was. I even went and bought new workout clothes after that class," chuckled Susan.

Before you head for the gym, face reality at home

We tend to avoid having pictures of us taken when we're heavy. And we rarely stand and stare at ourselves in a mirror either. Why? Because we don't want to see *what we know we look like*.

But most gyms have mirrors, and it will be far easier to confront yourself in your mirror alone at home, than when you are standing in a room exercising with everybody else... including those "everybodies" that are already in 2nd and 3rd gear.

But the truth is you already know how your clothes fit, which ones you're not wearing. Which ones you're pushing to the side of the closet for "some day when I'm slim again." But avoiding reality will only keep you stuck where you are, the size and health you are.

It takes two points to navigate a ship or a weight loss/health gain program. You must know *exactly where you are* and *exactly where you want to be*. So as you begin, take a good close look at your body and lovingly experience it *as it is*. This is your exact starting point... the point you'll look back to with pleasure in a few months. This is where you are as you start.

Take a good hard look!

Before you go stare at yourself in a mirror at the gym, stand in front of a mirror in your home. Take a few minutes to get comfortable looking at yourself. As you stare at your body, ask yourself what signals it has been sending you. Is it your breath, your posture or knees? Is it your energy, stamina or blood sugar levels? Is it your focus or mood?

What else have you noticed but ignored? Have you been avoiding bathing suits, pools and beaches? Putting off buying new clothes or getting dressed up for special occasions? Or avoiding looking for a job or relationship because of your body? Or avoiding creating goals and taking steps toward them? Are you depressed about your weight, health and life... even a little? You created getting here. Start creating where you want your body to be in six months or a year.

Don't expect to be racing along in 2nd gear when you start. You'll get there, but you'll have to begin slowly. You'll have to move through your fears and resistance. You'll have to learn the basics in 1st gear. And you will need a teacher beside you as you learn.

My 1st gear teacher was Mahara

An Israeli friend of mine invited me to go to his yoga class. Immediately I cringed at my image of people sitting Indian-style in a circle surrounded by the smell of incense and the sound of people chanting Ommmm. My friend said, Celso, you will be in for a surprise. Your ideas are really off-base!

We pulled up in a strip mall to an ordinary-looking storefront and stepped into an empty room, mirrored up front, and looking for-all-the-world like a gym. The class was a 90 minute workout that was far more strenuous than any gym workout I had ever done, and the heat added another challenging element. So if you have the same Ommmm image in your mind about hot sweaty yoga, it's time for you to update too.

The first time I met Mahara, she was teaching my class. She explained the benefits of each posture and how to do it correctly. She walked over to guide me as I struggled to get my stiff, awkward arms and legs into the right positions and reminded me to breathe through my nose which made me realize I had been gasping for air through my mouth. She showed me how to stand so I wouldn't hurt my back or put too much pressure on my knees. Having Mahara demonstrate each posture, let me progress more easily and safely. Her input was vital in 1st gear because I could have hurt myself without it.

Jesse and I invited Mahara for holiday meals so we not only heard about her way of eating but we got to see it in action. She selected healthy items and simply left the others alone. Mahara would always bring lots of fresh fruits and vegetables to add to our feast. She allowed us to understand her diet from her example.

Age doesn't matter, Mahara always said. No matter what age she is, age certainly doesn't matter to Mahara. She is flexible and has the kind of crazy stamina I could only have wished for then, but it's the kind of crazy stamina I have today. And I hope to keep until I am the one saying age doesn't matter!

Without realizing it, I could see that Susan was correct again. Mahara was my 1st gear teacher and if it were not for her, I probably would have given up on yoga after the first class... and given up on improving my diet as well.

How to succeed in 1st gear

In 1st gear, you need to have confidence in your leader and do what you are told, the way you are told to do it as long as you take care of yourself in the process. Sounds like childhood, doesn't it? In a lot of ways it is so *most adults avoid 1st gear like the plague.* They don't read manuals or online help files. They try to put together toys or bookshelves without looking at instruction sheets. They don't slow down to ask questions or listen to answers. But that's exactly what you will need to do *at this point in your weight losing/health gaining adventure.*

Remember what Susan said to me at our first meeting, "As we begin, you will need to set aside the rabbi part of you. That is *not* the part I will be coaching. You need to be open to learning and changing."

Susan's words mean a whole lot more to me now. And what she didn't say at the beginning, because I wouldn't have understood it then, was... Celso, you are in the 1st gear of learning the 10 success skills so you need to *be able to not know* at this stage."

Cracking "The Success Gear Code"
Word Cues to 1st gear

"Here are some words that tell you when you are in, or someone else is, in 1st gear:

right/wrong, good/bad, should/shouldn't, have to/must, always/never, safe/dangerous, correct/incorrect, dependent, needy, insecure, scared, worried, doubtful, nervous, hesitant, anxious, frightened, fearful, trying, pleasing, obedient and loyal.

Be patient with yourself. 1st gear is the toughest phase of success. Day after day, completion by completion, you're catching on. You may have setbacks, of course, but with some additional instruction you can begin again and succeed at a higher level. Your teacher is preparing you to shift into 2nd gear independence.

In the 2nd gear of success you become more efficient

The 2nd gear of success is for doing more-better-faster, for meeting and exceeding specific values and standards, for competing against your own performance and other's.

In 2nd gear, you want to begin working more independently. Your teacher is no longer there all the time and you're glad of course, but now you need to start noticing each sign of improvement. Each old pound lost. Each new flexibility gained. Each fatty area reduced. You need to be responsible for your success and self-confidence.

I am clearly in 2nd gear in Bikram now. I know how to safely do all 26 postures and each time I do them I get better... more precise, more relaxed and strong. Instead of struggling and hesitating, I am confident and certain. I know the sequence by heart and I'm enjoying pushing my limits.

You need to Success File for yourself in 2nd gear

In 2nd gear, daily Success Filing is essential. Without it, internal resistance will overtake you as you work to do more-better-faster. And more-better-faster still. You'll be tired and sore sometimes. You'll want to skip a walk, class or workout. You'll start using all the tried-and-true excuses that used to work for you. But not this time. This time you're committed to losing weight and gaining health.

In 2nd gear you need to take responsibility for adding to Your Success File. To succeed in 2nd gear, you can no longer be other-confident. *You must constantly work not just on your workout but on building your self-confidence as well.*

On good days and bad days, you will need to keep your desired outcome in mind. In my case, seeing my daughter Sophie enjoying having me there with her at her wedding someday... something I missed! In Susan's case, full use of her knee.

Susan's health challenge was different than mine. Hers wasn't weight. It was mobility. She had had a serious knee injury and her orthopedic surgeon told her it was inoperable. "Learn to live with it!" But Susan simply laughed, "That's not an option" and she set out on her own path of healing. Today her knee is working far better than before the injury. I know because I exercise beside her!

Word Cues to 2nd gear

Here are some words that will signal when you or your teacher is shifting into 2nd gear: more-better-faster, more repetitions, more stretch and extension, more exertion, more flexibility, more sweat, more strength, more endurance. In the business world, 2nd gear also includes words like win/lose, better/worse, quantity/quality, competition, hard work, deadlines, burnout, injuries, scores, charts, graphs, quotas, bonuses, raises, prizes, plaques, promotions, stress and disease," explained Susan.

Susan is in 2nd gear in Bikram but 3rd gear in other areas of her life

"I'm not in the 3rd gear of Bikram yet. But here's what 3rd gear is like in other areas of my life.

When I was designing my jungle home, I regularly woke up in the night full of new ideas. I couldn't sleep because there were so many images in my head. I was excited, asking questions, doing research, sketching and planning. I shared what I had in mind in great detail with my contractor giving him an accurate picture, soundtrack and feeling. Answering his questions in as much detail as possible. Asking him what it will take to construct what I had in mind, the cost in time and materials. Making him a co-dreamer and a co-creator, working together day by day, step by step. Celebrating our results together, walking across the bamboo bridge, tip toeing along the black-river-rock path. Taking long steps across the stepping stones to the banana jungle, past the new water lilies and sea lettuces. Yes, that's why they call me, Jungle Mama.

Word cues to 3rd gear

These words tell you when you have shifted into 3rd gear: aha, excitement, spontaneity, creativity, realization, flexibility, simplicity, ease, cooperation, communication, caring, compassion, sensitivity, satisfaction and fulfillment.

In the business world, it also includes words like teamwork, mission, service, health, balance, holistic, healing, integrity, choice and ease. When you hear yourself using words like these, you'll know you have shifted into the 3rd gear of success in exercise, at work or in life," concluded Susan.

Remember, when your Success File is full, you feel success-full. When it is low, you feel dependent and needy, unsure and insecure. Afraid to move ahead in new areas.

Ok, back to my story. I always hated exercise. I never knew why it was so difficult for me. In 2006, I developed sleep apnea. I couldn't get more than a couple of hours of RAM sleep a night... and neither could Jesse. I tried the CPAP machine but it was like having the turbine of an airplane blowing on my nose as I attempted to sleep.

I hated exercise until I figured out why

My doctor told me there was a surgery he could do that would remove part of my soft pallet, tonsils and uvula, (The uvula is the little dangling flesh in the back of your mouth) I said yes.

When he was performing the surgery, he was amazed by what he saw. He called the other doctors over to look. They couldn't believe it either. I had the smallest air passage they had ever seen. They said it was the same size as a baby's. The surgery was supposed to take 45 minutes but it took five hours.

He said that tight air passage was what made exercising so hard for me. I simply couldn't get enough air to work out. After that I started losing weight far more easily. But my doctor warned me that if I gained my weight back, that air passage would close up again and I'd be back exactly where I was. I listened and changed. I've kept my 100 pounds off and now every breath I take during exercise is a pleasure.

Look out... injuries frequently occur in 2nd gear!

In 1st gear you need to follow the rules so you can learn safely and correctly. But in 2nd gear your approach shifts. The goal of 2nd gear is doing more-better-faster and more-better-faster still. You push against your limits and sometimes your body pushes back. Increased productivity becomes more important than safety... at least for a while.

After working out at the gym for a month, I felt confident enough to begin increasing the amount of weight I was lifting. Each time I added additional weight I took a few days to acclimate.

After a year, I was lifting 40 pounds more than my weight and headed higher, until I woke up one morning with a shooting pain in my right shoulder. I went to see my doctor and he told me that it was probably a torn rotator cuff. He recommended that I see an orthopedic surgeon and a neurologist. But first I went to my gym, found a personal trainer and explained my situation to him.

If I had gone to a doctor he probably would have given me steroids to cover up the pain and I might have continued working out and injuring myself more. That is what "the old me" would have done, but this time I was committed to finding a way to work through my injury and I did.

My new trainer got the picture right away. He knew far more than I did. He told me to work with free weights instead of a fixed bar. He said the fixed bar causes this sort of injury because it doesn't allow the muscles to move freely and readapt when you're pressing too hard.

He explained that in the U.S. we spend hours bent forward over our computer, mouse in our hand with our arms rotated internally. As a result lots of people suffer from carpal tunnel pain. After work, we go to the gym and do chest presses, shoulder presses, pushups, with our arms rotated in again. The outcome? Supraspinatus tendonitis, an overuse injury of the rotator cuff.

He told me rowing with cables is an excellent way to externally rotate your arms and balance your shoulders. Here, Rabbi, grab the cables in front of you and pull your arms back, rotating your palms away and behind you. It felt strange at first but after a few repetitions it became more comfortable and familiar.

I had to scale back my exercise program for a couple of weeks so I could let my shoulder rest and heal. That was the toughest part for me. During that recovery period I worked on developing my core strength and I had to shift back into 1st gear. I had not worked this area of my body before and I had to slow myself down enough to learn.

After six weeks, my pain was gone despite the fact that many people told me it would take at least six months. When you pay attention to what is creating the pain and change what you are doing, your body will miraculously heal itself.

During those painful weeks, I learned to be more patient. And I was reminded again...health and safety come first in 1st gear!

Proceed slowly in 1st gear

"Trying to start your car in 2nd or 3rd gear doesn't work. Accelerating too quickly in 2nd gear doesn't work either. Slow down, gear down, ask questions and follow directions until you understand why your teachers are providing the instructions they are, until you have the knowledge and experience to make good and safe choices without their constant supervision, feedback and acknowledgment. Until you can avoid painful injuries and time-consuming setbacks.

Whether it's yoga or an alligator farm, you need to master the basics first! In hindsight, your father's words... go to school and learn more about alligators first... was excellent advice!

We spent most of our time in 1st gear in childhood, in school and at home, learning what others expected us to do and when to do it. And we built up lots of resistance. Yes, that's the reason most adults avoid learning new things! They hate the old feelings they get in 1st gear. They hate being told what to do. They hate feeling dependent and ignorant. They hate following directions. But, like it or not, gearing down into 1st gear is what you will need to do to succeed at new routines, new shopping lists , new foods, new exercise programs and, soon as a bonus, you'll be meeting new people and making new friends!" exclaimed Susan.

Start with walking. Walking is really good exercise!

If you weigh 200 pounds and you walk briskly for 45 minutes, you can burn 351 calories! Compare that to golfing with an electric cart for 45 minutes which only burns 234 calories. Or running for 45 minutes which burns 576!

No, I can't run for 45 minutes but I can walk for an hour and a half and burn 702 calories. So I walk more, park farther away from the mall and take stairs instead of elevators or escalators.

Easy work outs you can do while watching TV

Exercise during commercials instead of heading for the refrigerator! Start with 10 pushups, then 15 and 20. I do a series of about 100 now. You can do sit ups or squats while watching TV too. I even use my daughter Sophie as a weight, having her climb on my back and hold on while I do pushups.

Nobody likes being the fat person in the gym!

And I didn't either. But as soon as I began losing weight and gaining definition, working out became a high for me. My body was producing endorphins which block pain perception, and serotonin which makes you feel happy! In fact, it's sometimes called "the happy hormone" even though it's not really a hormone at all.

How flexible are you?

How flexible are you not just in your body but in your mind and your habits? Have you become resistant to change, only willing to do what you have already done, familiar things?

Simple questions to ask yourself but the answers are not easy. I found rigid parts of me as soon as I began changing my diet and exercise! And so will you. But press through so you can enjoy a new body and life. Susan and I know. We did it and so can you!

OK, it's time to take your Before Shot

Take a few minutes to snap a photo of you. Shorts and a top or a bathing suit are the best things to wear. *Tell your phone or camera the truth!* No one has to see this shot now! But we're sure you'll want to show it in the days to come! Or add it to our website in a few months... www.codreamsuccess.com.

Next dig around in your photo drawer or scrapbook and find some old pictures of you. Were you slim then? Or were you heavy then too? Is this a return or a revolution?

Place your picture on the refrigerator door or your bathroom mirror or wherever else you pass frequently. Or if you can't confront it right now, bury it in the bottom of your underwear drawer for a month or two.

This is your starting point... your Before Shot. A picture you'll look back to with pride, pleasure and inspiration in just a few months!

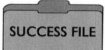

SUCCESS FILE

Time to Success File again...
Diet Skill Three: Shifting Gears... starting, accelerating and creating your weight loss

Here are a few successes to get you started...
drank lots of water
took my first yoga class and made it all the way through!
was able to stare at myself in the mirror and feel OK
remembered how I used to feel when I was fit, it inspired me!
plan to go Monday, Wednesday and Friday mornings
noticed 1st gear word cues my instructor or trainer was using
felt sore and went Wed anyway... a little easier
understood what to do better, teacher was really helpful
getting used to planning food, taking snacks and water
found someone to walk with who lives nearby
can actually see myself getting slim and fit now!
noticed work call was filled with 2nd gear word cues and stresses
took my before picture and looked through old photographs
remembered being made fun of in gym class as a kid
may have a new codreamer who just started losing weight
met our contractor and shifted to 3rd gear, amazing to see gears!
planning weekend, where to eat and what activity to do
went food shopping and was able to get new foods more easily
bought meat and vegetables to make kabobs on the grill
got recommendations for healthy foods and restaurants
cooked fish filet with greens on top... really easy, tasted great!

Diet Skill Four: Hologramming... how to get what you want far more easily

"Like a computer, your brain has a search function. But unlike a computer, it searches *instantly and unconsciously* 24 hours a day, seven days a week! What does it search for? It searches for what you have in mind... positive or negative, like it or not," explained Susan.

"Your Reticular Activating System, or Razz as I call it, is a bundle of nerve fibers at the base of your brain. Your Razz alerts you when *sensory data coming in through your eyes, ears, nose, taste buds or muscles* matches the *sensory data of a plan or dream you have imagined.*

For example, if you tell yourself you need toothpaste, then the next time you're in the grocery store walking down the aisle, toothpaste will come to mind. 'Oh, yeah, I need toothpaste.' And you reach out, put it in your cart and avoid another trip to the store.

Is your Razz working for you, or against you?

Your Razz is the part of your brain that alerts you in the night when something you planned has been left incomplete. Have you ever found yourself lying awake in bed in a panic? I was supposed to but I didn't. Oh no! I forgot. Whether it's to mail your taxes, call your mom or buy healthy groceries. That was your Razz urging you to take action now.

Have you ever seen holograms? Did you see Star Wars?

What is your Razz searching for 24/7? It is searching for sensory data that matches holographic brain recordings you have created or... to say it quickly... it is searching for holograms.

Most of us have seen holograms at Disney World, in science museums or on credit cards. Some holograms appear to swell in or out three dimensionally. Others appear as volumetric images in space, like R2D2's hologram of Princess Leia pleading for galactic assistance in *Star Wars*.

Your brain creates holographic recordings whenever you think, plan or dream

Dr. Karl Pribram, Nobel nominee and *The Einstein of Brain Research* says memories are recorded holographically… whole in each cell.

Holograms are created using two or more laser beams. Holographic brain recordings are created using two or more laser-like inputs from your senses—seeing, hearing, feeling, tasting, smelling, touching and doing.

When data coming in through your senses matches a holographic recording… like buy toothpaste or fresh fruit, thank John or share a possible solution with your carpenter, your Razz alerts you. Zap! Stop, look and listen. The opportunity to take a step toward completing, deleting or creating a hologram you have in mind is nearby!

Have you ever wondered why some people seem to regularly get what they want while others seldom do? Some people are doing a different sort of thinking or dreaming. Consciously or unconsciously they are using a method I call Hologramming.

When you imagine what you want to experience in as much detail as possible, its color and shape, its size and weight, its sound and movement, its texture, emotions and feelings, when you pre-experience living it, you create a holographic recording of that outcome in your brain. A set of *detailed* specifications your Razz then begins to search and alert you to opportunities," said Susan.

A Masters Degree in Design

In retrospect, one of the smartest things I ever did was get a Masters Degree in interior design. Why? Because to earn that degree, I had to get really good at hologramming.

My professors called it visualizing, but it wasn't just visualizing, it was pre-experiencing the homes I was designing and hologramming them in action. Where do you enter and where do you leave? Where does the plumbing go and how about the electrical? What is the flow of movement through the house? What happens when it snows or rains? When it's sunny and hot? And on and on, I had to be able to see, hear, feel, taste and even smell the home and family that would live in it, morning, noon and night.

I remember getting vicious headaches when I first began to design. I had never pressed myself to get that clear or that detailed before. But that's what we all have to teach ourselves to do if we want to experience the weight and health we have in mind... if we want to live our holograms. To anticipate our need for healthy snacks, to understand calories, fats and sodium content so we can make healthy choices, to teach ourselves to like the foods our bodies like and need.

When we understand more about our body and more about nutrition, we won't need other people to lay out diets for us, and go on and off of them. We will be able to create our own food and exercise plan day-by-day, circumstance-by-circumstance.

The more detail, the more power

According to Dr. Pribram, some thoughts are more powerful than others. *To increase the power of your thoughts, you must think in great detail and use all your senses.* You need to see them, hear them, feel them, even taste and smell them.

Bottom line... the more detail, the more power.

Your thoughts and the forcefield they generate are *the steering mechanism for your life*

If you use this attractive forcefield positively, it can increase the probability of your getting what you want. Slimmer and healthier. But if you use it negatively, it can increase the probability of getting what you dread! Sick, ill or alone. Your thoughts and the forcefield they generate are *the steering mechanism of your life.*

Our holographic recordings are what we call memory

Everything you have ever experienced is recorded holographically in your brain, every picture you've ever seen, every sound you've heard, every feeling you've sensed, every taste, every smell... everything. No, you don't have conscious access to every holographic recording, but every once in a while a whole cluster of them will pop into your mind and body. Bam! And you are there," smiled Susan.

I almost drowned

When I was four, I fell in a pool and nearly drowned. I remember hitting the water, breathing it in and filling up my lungs. I remember seeing bubbles escaping from my mouth and a cigarette floating down toward me. It was the once-lit cigarette my Dad had in his mouth when he dove in to save me. That holographic memory raises hairs on my arms to this today!

Your holographic memories are stored in your brain in living sound and color, complete with everything you have ever felt and done. Whether you remember them consciously or you retrieve them through hypnosis, your holographic memory gives you access to everything you have experienced... *and pre-experienced*. Yes, pre-experienced too! Every plan or dream you have created for the future.

Think Miami, Think Thai

When Jesse and I lived in Mississippi and flew to Miami to visit our families, our mouths started watering as soon as our plane started to descend. Jesse and I had a ritual. When we deplaned, we would always head for Thai food at Siam River. It was close to where we were staying and open late at night. We knew someday Miami would be our home and we were so happy to be there that I would find myself literally hugging the steering wheel. Yes, Miami is where we live today. A completion success for us both!

We loved the atmosphere of Siam River. It was dimly lit and causal. The servers were dressed in traditional silky Thai-wrapped attire. We would take off our shoes, sit on the floor, lean comfortably against triangular red and gold Thai bolsters and order our favorites... Stand-Up Chicken and Mango with Sticky Rice. We ate there whenever we came to Miami and whenever we left.

What is disappointment... really?

"But what if Siam River were closed for some reason? And there were no dimly lit room with servers in traditional silky Thai-wrapped attire? No Stand-Up Chicken or Mango with Sticky Rice? No satisfaction for your Thai-watering mouths?

Disappointment is holographic too. *We're disappointed when what we see, hear, feel, smell and taste doesn't match the hologram we have in mind*, whether it's a long-anticipated gift, a first kiss or Thai food in Miami.

Oh, no. That isn't what I had in mind. *A holographic mismatch*, an empty feeling. Oh man, I'm disappointed.

When you're stressed, upset, worried, disappointed, sad or depressed? What do you eat, drink and do then? Sweet, salty, alcoholic, spicy or other? How else can you deal with these feelings? It's time to create new holograms that will allow you to lose weight and gain health... no matter what, where or when. Life goes on even when you're on a diet.

Marketers understand your holographic brain too!

There's a giant food industry out there working to get you hooked on *what they make and profit from,* even though it's not necessarily what you need and want. Yes, manufacturers create holograms too and they are very, very multi-sensory and detailed!

Major brands pay to have their well-constructed holograms repeated over and over on TV, on signs, on buses, by mail and on the internet, presented to you in full brilliant color with lively, appealing soundtracks as well! They spend billions of dollars to come up with ways to convince you to buy their holograms, instead of yours.

If you go into a store without a detailed plan in mind, *the detailed plan they have in mind for you* will probably win out. Remember the more detail, the more power a hologram has.

Their plan is to sell you salty, sugary, highly-processed, low-cost, high-profit products. And to hook you on them so you will need to come back and buy more. Is your plan or list detailed enough to withstand their billion-dollar holographic power? Will you walk out of the store with what you came in wanting? Or with what they want you to buy? Will they seduce you with coupons or special offers that will make it seem like a too-good-to-pass-up deal?

The products on your list will be what you pay for at the checkout and put in your cabinet and refrigerator, in your body or your family's bodies... if your hologram is highly detailed. More highly detailed than theirs! And the extra products you buy will probably be because of their professionally-built holograms

Drug stores... candy up front, diabetic supplies in back

We've talked about grocery stores and fast food restaurants. But how about drug stores, are they promoting health or profit?

Drug stores get you coming and going. The front of a drug store offers you candy and snack foods. And what's in the back? Go look for yourself. I noticed this when my husband Albert was diagnosed with diabetes and we had to purchase a meter to test his blood sugar. The prescription area is surrounded with diabetes supplies... meters, strips, lancets and meal substitutes. *If you buy what they sell up front, you'll need to buy what they sell in back.* Yes, if you are unconscious, drugstores will get you coming and going.

Red alert! Temptation Days... holidays and memories

Think Thanksgiving, think food. Think birthday, think food. Think weddings, anniversaries and graduations. Think Hanukah, Christmas and New Years. Think food. Bar Mitzvahs and Christenings. Food and more food and more food.

Every food sets off a cascade of multi-sensory memories. Memories of tastes, smells, occasions, celebrations. All the times you ate food for pleasure.

When you access these memories they will make you want to eat these pleasure-associated foods again... unless you have an even stronger *positive holographic future* in mind, an even stronger image of your body and health. And codreamers who have your hologram in mind too.

But before your next Temptation Days stop and think. Why do you celebrate these occasions? What do they really mean to you? Thanksgiving, birthdays, anniversaries and graduations. Hanukah, Christmas and New Years. How can you celebrate these life events differently? With new experiences or menus, healthier foods and drinks?

Take time to create and pre-experience new holograms for these special days... ones that will enhance your health and longevity, not put on extra pounds you'll have to work for weeks to take off.

Be on alert on bad memory days too... days of big life events, losses, divorces, disappointments. Days you may be tempted to use food to comfort yourself. To stuff or drown your feelings," warned Susan.

Susan asked me to share a detailed, multisensory hologram of how I changed my approach to travel and food. Enjoy this story, detail by detail. Read it actively, seeing, hearing, feeling, tasting and smelling what he is sharing so you can experience it too.

I planned my trips around food

Each summer, I travel the world organizing retreats and speaking to large audiences. Before I lost weight, I used to plan all my trips around food. I was obsessed from the moment I left home. Worried about what I would do if I got hungry in the night, I stopped by a duty free shop at the airport and stocked up on chocolates to have as my stash on the plane and at my hotel.

I was a food-traveler as well as a world-traveler. I researched restaurants where I wanted to go. I have eaten in the palace in Beijing where Peking Duck was created. I had pho in Vietnam in the same Ho Chi Min restaurant where Bill Clinton had eaten. I enjoyed Mexican food at George Bush's favorite spot in Texas, ate at The Ivy among celebrities in L.A., and dined at hot spots in European capitals. I was a food-provider-manufacturer-and travel-guide advertiser's dream come true! But no more.

I reset my internal GPS

Today I am lighter and I travel lighter too! I check into my hotel, find a grocery store, buy fruit, fresh juices and nuts, and then I take a long walk to explore my new area. I wander through street markets and check out events and neighborhoods off the beaten path. I talk to people and I am invited into their homes and lives. My new approach to food makes my traveling experience far richer and more enlivening than dressing up for exotic meals, paying sometimes over 100 Euros per person and having acid reflux all night!

On my last trip to Berlin, 95 pounds lighter, I headed out for my exploratory walk. The scenery was magnificent-- the shops, the bridges, people coming home from work, calling their children to come in for dinner. I was enjoying a slice of their lives when I suddenly realized I had walked 20 miles and I was hungry! Fortunately I found myself in an ethnic neighborhood and I ordered Vietnamese food, fresh, beautiful, and nutritious. And it only cost five Euros.

Interestingly enough I still remember how that simple Vietnamese meal tasted, but I simply can't remember what I ate in those fancy, expensive restaurants. It was more about place and celebrities than enjoying God's miraculous food and nutrition. The details of my holographic food memories are no longer attractive to me and they no longer unconsciously pull me in their direction. I have reset my GPS!

Now instead of seeing the world from inside restaurants, I see it from outside, from streets and towers, gardens and museums, theaters and dancing. Even the photographs I take are different. They are pictures of fresh vegetables in the market, the view from a castle tower I visited, or the top of the Pyramid of the Sun at Teotihuacan after I climbed up all those high steps to the top, or of a kids' bubble festival in Berlin. Savoring these new views is fantastically liberating and delicious at a whole new level!

A wise man once told me that happiness is a measure of how few things enslave you. I am happy now that I have one less thing enslaving me! Food. It is clear that what was holding me back was not my stomach but my mind.

What you think is what you get, like it or not
"Here's the bottom line... What you think is what you get, like it or not. So think about *what you do want* instead of *what you*

don't want. And believe it or not, "thinking about *what you do want*" can make the difference between life and death!

Physicians are discovering that *looking forward to* is essential to your health. Surgeons in my *Technology of Success* seminars told me stories about patients who, going in for surgery with next-to-no chance of survival, pulled through miraculously. They had a hologram to live for—seeing their daughter graduate from college, holding their first grandchild, moving into the nearly-finished home they had dreamed of for years. And they lived to experience what they had hologrammed for so long in so much detail.

Those same surgeons also told me stories about very depressed patients who, in for minor surgeries, died on the table. They seemed to have given up on dreaming—and living!

Adults who had their dreams squashed as kids and adults, who have been disappointed over and over, sometimes try to prevent more pain by giving up on dreaming. But they don't realize that, when they limit their dreaming, they limit their success.

On his TV show *New York Med* cardiothoracic surgeon Dr. Oz said he won't operate on a patient who doesn't have a loved one nearby. In big moments, we all need people beside us who care. Our health and well-being depend on it.

Which holograms is your Razz searching for? Yours or other peoples'

Remember, your Razz is searching for what you have in mind 24/7. But which holograms do you want your Razz to alert you about... holograms from your past... your familiar overeating habits, your old fears and upsets? Or holograms for your future...

your new ways of eating and exercising, your new body and life? *Razz notifications happen in an instant, but they can impact your feelings and actions for hours!" stated Susan.*

When I was still addicted to food, every afternoon at 2:00 when my blood sugar was low, I would suddenly start imagining eating Chinese food. My senses would fill up with vivid holographic memories! I could see it, feel it, smell it even feel my mouth filling up with saliva as if I were chewing it. And like a robot, I would head out the door to go buy it!

Conflicting holograms... you need to do some cleaning out

Chinese food or weight loss, you need to take some time to sort through your holograms, your old ones and your current ones. Which ones do you want your Razz to alert you about now? Which ones have a higher priority?

Was I using another one of the 10 success skills?

Susan asked me how I resisted those powerful, mouth-watering past holograms? And the minute she asked, I realized that instead of continuing to focus on eating on Chinese food, I had switched holograms. I started focusing on my body and health instead and what I needed to do became crystal clear and I headed for the gym.

Choose your direction... back to overeating or ahead to a new body and life

Moment-to-moment, you must choose. You can continue to focus on what you used to eat and head for your car. Or you can switch to your new hologram of the slim trim "future you" and head for your workout. *The hologram you focus on will determine the direction you go... back to overeating or ahead to new life.*

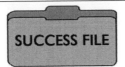

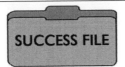

SUCCESS FILE

Time to Success File again.
Diet Skill Four: Hologramming
The more detail, the more power

List 3 holograms you want to make more detailed and powerful, like 1. the weight, size and fitness level you will be enjoying, what you arms will look like, your abs, your new flexibility and ease of movement. 2. the relationship you want to be enjoying, what you will be doing and where will you will be going together. 3. How your weight loss will be impacting your life and children's lives. What will they be feeling and doing differently as a result of your changes? Or anything else that really matters to you.

Now pre-live each future experience in as much detail as possible... see it, hear it, feel it, even taste it and smell it. Make sure *you step into the scene* and enjoy it, not just watch it from the wings! Once you pre-live it, it will be programmed in your Razz so your brain can alert you when opportunities are at hand!

Have you noticed holograms other people have programmed into your mind... parents, teachers, bosses, manufacturers or advertisers? Which of them do you want to update or delete?

Do you have more than one hologram for the same thing? You need to choose. Which one do you really want?

Turn to the back of the book now and add as many more Successes as you can.

Diet Skill Five: Switching... The Alchemy of Success, how to turn negatives into gold

When HSPs are stuck in negative they ask themselves, what do I want instead?

Susan, I remember what you said the day we started working together. You told me you were sure I was using all 10 success skills, but I wasn't sure. Let's see which ones you have used so far. First is Success Filing. Second is Updating. Third is Shifting Gears. Fourth is Hologramming. And now I realize that I have been using the fifth success skill as well, Switching.

Ten skills, Susan? We're at five and headed in the right direction! OK, let's keep going!

"Yes, Celso, unfortunately your Razz acts *just as powerfully in negative as in positive*! Whenever you encounter new situations your brain *instantaneously and unconsciously* searches your memory. What happened last time? What does this look, sound, feel, taste and smell like?

Did I succeed before or did I fail? Did I get hurt? Was I disappointed? Should I avoid this situation? Or should I take action? All this decision-making happens in a fraction of a second! And it happens unconsciously.

Yes, that experience might be something you *should have avoided* when you were younger and far less experienced! Something you should have feared. But now it is something vital for you to do!

Making the impossible, possible

Have you ever noticed that the most wonderful things in life may have seemed impossible at the start... like finding a mate, getting a job, buying a home, going to school, raising a child or losing 100 pounds?

There are *two ways of living... focused on successes, past and future. Or focused on failures*, past and future, and letting your Survival Brain force you to constantly re-live and pre-live those old failures and disappointments! Remember *re* means past, re-vive, re-call, re-discover, re-do, re-new! And *pre* means *future*, pre-view, pre-experience and pre-celebrate!

What you think is what you get, like it not. Yes, positive or negative, past or future, you have a choice! But sadly you don't always exercise that choice! *Using your creative brain positively is the most important exercise program of all!*

The Positive Command Brain... your brain *only* operates in positive

Stop for a minute and think about what *your brain only operates in positive* really means. If you put a negative word--*not, but, can't, shouldn't, impossible, never*-- in a sentence, the hologram stays *the same. Don't think about chocolate* equals *think about chocolate* to the brain!" added Susan.

A Positive Command Brain, yes, this makes sense to me now. When you tell me I can't eat something, that's exactly what I want. During Passover when I can't have bread, I want bread far more than during the rest of the year.

"Negative words simply create resistance, anxiety, worry and stress in your mind and body. Why? Because you are using your Positive Command Brain incorrectly! Those feelings signal that you need to *change the way you are thinking*. Switch to positive.

You need to see, hear, feel, taste, smell and say *what you do want* so your Miraculous Brain can work correctly and easily.

I once read about a language in which every word was positive. They always said what they wanted and what they meant. I can only imagine how much more efficient that language would be for getting what you want... how many more goals you would be able to achieve. And how much more responsible that language would force us to be!

Program your Razz instead of letting others program it for you

When you imagine your goals and dreams in detail, your miraculous brain searches for opportunities and zaps you... OK, here it is! Here is something you have in mind... a new meal idea, a new exercise program, someone to exercise with, a new approach like eating thermogenic foods, Raspberry Ketone or *Conquer The Fat-Loss Code*...or whatever else might move you in the direction you want to go. Then it will be up to you to test it out. It's time to focus on what you do want instead of *what you don't want*! You are a powerful creator. A co-creator with God!" affirmed Susan.

FDA head resorted to dumpster diving!

Dr. David Kessler, a medical school dean and former commissioner of the Food and Drug Administration, had an addiction similar to mine... Kessler's was Chili's Southwestern Eggrolls and Boneless Shanghai Wings. The man in him wanted to eat them, and the scientist in him wanted to know why. But unlike foods in grocery stores, foods in restaurants are not required to have Nutrition Labels so he was on a mission to discover what the mouth-watering treats he was addicted to actually contained.

"He went in the middle of the night, long after the last employee had locked up the Chili's Grill and Bar. He'd steer his car around the back, check to make sure no one was around and then quietly approach the dumpster," wrote Lyndsey Layton of *The Washington Post*[19]. "If anyone noticed the man foraging through the trash, they would have assumed he was a vagrant. Except he was wearing black dress slacks and padded gardening gloves. 'I'm surprised he didn't wear a tie,' his wife said dryly."

Sometimes he would reach in and poke around from the outside of the dumpster but sometimes he climbed inside. What was driving this nattily-dressed man to such extreme behavior?

The Addictive Mix... salt, fat and sugar!

He wanted to find empty boxes with ingredient labels that would reveal what ingredients Chili's uses to make the Southwestern Eggrolls, Boneless Shanghai Wings and other dishes they serve. And he did. "The labels showed the foods were bathed in salt, fat and sugars, beyond what a diner might expect by reading the menu," Kessler said.[20]

Salt appeared eight times. Various sugars five times. These tasty appetizers, filled with chopped chicken to make them faster to eat, are deep fried. So despite their small size and innocent appearance, these egg rolls contained 910 calories, 57 grams of fat and 1,960 milligrams of sodium!

Our brains and our children's brains are being captured by fast foods!

Kessler revealed his startling theory in his book, *The End of Overeating*. "Much of the scientific research around overeating has been physiology -- what's going on in our body," he said. "The real question is what's going on in our brain. And the food industry manipulates this neurological response, designing foods to induce people to eat more than they should or even want. The challenge is how do we explain to America what's going on -- how do we break through and help people understand how their brains have been captured?" Kessler said."

If you don't know what YOU want, you'll probably get what somebody else wants

And that somebody seems to be the food and drug producers of the world! They have food engineers and high-powered marketers who are paid billions to manipulate your mind and purchases... think about child-oriented ads on TV, for example. Fruit Loops and Pop Tarts, Doritos and Cokes. But stop for a second. You can create powerful, highly-detailed holograms, too, and take back your power!

Returning to *The Miracle Diet*... the natural proportion of sugar, fat, salt and calories

You have a choice. You can continue eating the foods manufacturers want you to buy that are making you unhealthy. Or you can return to eating the foods God provided for you, already magnificently packaged in their own skins, rinds, pods and shells. Foods that contain all the human-appropriate vitamins and minerals you need, *and the right proportion of sugar, fat, salt and calories.* Will you listen to God, or will you continue listening to the marketing and advertising gurus whose agenda has nothing to do with your health?

We pray for health and God answers. But do we listen?

There is no clergy on earth that hasn't told this story at least once. But it's a good and highly relevant, so here goes. A man in a flood climbed up on his roof and asked God to rescue him. Soon a man in a boat came and offered to save him. He said No. God is coming to save me so the man in the boat left. Next a helicopter flew over, dropped a ladder and told the man to climb up. Again he told the man No that God is coming to save him so the helicopter left too. Finally the water rose so high that the man was forced to swim and swim until he was so exhausted that he drowned.

After death, he met God and asked why He did not save him. To which God calmly answered, I sent you a boat and a helicopter and you refused both my efforts.

Don't be the guy who dies and goes to heaven only to hear God say, I sent you all the fruits, vegetables and meats you need to be healthy, but instead you decided to eat fast food!

Hologramming... pre-experiencing yourself in great shape

To increase your diet and exercise power, stand in front of a mirror and pre-experience liking *the you* you see there! Your firm, muscular, flexible, healthy body.

Visualize yourself happily dressing for a special occasion and feeling excited about how you look and feel! Or visualize yourself doing aerobics, yoga or whatever exercise you choose and doing it easily and skillfully. Picture what you are wearing and how great you look in it. See yourself performing skillfully and proficiently, breathing smoothly and easily. Get excited and enthusiastic. That's the future you! Let *that you* attract you there.

One of the things I regret most in my life is that I spent so much time eating when I could have been doing other valuable things. Overeating is an addiction that costs lots of time and money. And costs your health too!

A secret Highly Successful People know... success has not one, but 3 essential parts!

"Now that you know more about your Miraculous Brain, let's review success and its 3 essential parts... completion, deletion and creation.

1-Success is completing holograms you have in mind

Success is realizing the details you are experiencing in reality match the details you have recorded in your Razz. Wow, I'm successful! This is exactly what I had in mind... or even better.

Yes, or even better! Whenever you realize this is *a match-plus*, you need to update your hologram! If you fail to update, you will miss the astounding gift your Miraculous Brain is offering... something even better than what you had imagined! I get chills whenever this happens! And yes, I'm starting to recognize these chills as a signal, a signal that something even better is right here in front of me.

2- Success is deleting outgrown holograms and replacing them with new ones

Success is deleting old holograms you have programmed in your memory, programmed *by you* or *for you by others*... parents, teachers, manufacturers, advertisers, movies and TV. Yes, movies and TV frequently shape the way we think we should look and what we think we should wear and buy! And even how we feel.

How do you delete a highly detailed, many times repeated hologram? *You replace it with a detailed, many times pre-experienced hologram of the new habits you want to develop,"* explained Susan.

For me it's enjoying frozen grapes and mangoes instead of ice cream. I look forward to these tastes just as much as I used to look forward to eating a pint of ice cream. Now I look back and tell myself, *a dessert is a dessert* whether it contains lots of sugar and fat, or fruit and fiber.

You can delete and replace places you used to eat or simply replace what you order from their menu. Instead of ordering steak, I order a chicken breast without skin. Instead of french fries, I order steamed or grilled vegetables. Instead of pizza, now we order sushi. That made a huge difference. It was not just pizza for dinner but there were lots of leftovers so we had it for two days not just one.

You can also delete and replace what you used to do to reduce stress, and reduce your weight at the same time, like going out for a long walk instead of eating a bag of potato chips in front of the TV.

I updated my travel-to-eat approach to my new travel-to-enjoy local people, places and unique foods approach. When I think about summer I don't think about fancy restaurants, rich desserts and celebrities. Instead I think about which local cultural events I can enjoy and which parks and festivals I can experience. And where I can go to savor fresh fruits native to that area... dragon fruit, rambutan or jaboticaba.

3- Success is creating exciting new holograms and updating them as you learn more and more

"Success is creating and pre-experiencing the holographic details of the new life you want. It's savoring those details over and over to increase their attractive power, to load them into your Razz so it can start alerting you when opportunities are at hand. Stop, look and listen! What you have in mind is close by!" exclaimed Susan.

New body, new life

What do you want to do that you haven't done because of your weight or health? What places do you want to see? What experiences do you want to have? Maybe it's as sky-high as taking a suborbital space flight. Or as far-flung as traveling to China or Tibet. Maybe it's announcing to your friends that you are ready to find a loving relationship. Or taking a course or finishing a degree. Or changing jobs or joining a sports team. Or learning to ballroom dance. Or to swim or dive, or anything else your heart desires.

New body, old closet!

It's time to rethink what's in your closet and your drawers. What do you have there that you really want to wear? And what is out-of-date and simply taking up space? Some dieters hang a "future outfit" on their closet door to inspire and motivate them... a powerful cause for celebration in the weeks to come when you try it on... and it fits! Perfectly.

Time to buy something new

Maybe it's time to buy something you really like. Even if you lose too much to wear it in a few months, you can always give it away or donate it. What would you like to wear? How would you like to look? What kind of relationship would you like to be in?

Think about it and *choose*. Yes, choose by pre-experiencing it in as much detail as possible. And step into it. Be there now, see it, hear it, feel it and enjoy it. Take back the creative power God has given you.

Here is an assignment for you...

Take a few minutes when you wake up, while you're eating breakfast or driving, to "future" or "pre-experience" the day you would like to live.

No, you can't make it turn out exactly the way you imagine, but you can increase the efficiency of your God-given Positive Command Brain and your Razz so that it can alert you to opportunities, people and connections you might otherwise walk right past... just like that toothpaste!

When I started my diet, I imagined running a mile. When I ran my first mile, I felt very accomplished. Very success-full. Today I run 3 miles! Maybe what's next for me is a marathon or a triathlon.

Other peoples' stories help you remember your own

This time, it's not a diet.

It's a new way of life, and you will need partners to succeed in this turnaround. You may not know who these people are now, but you will soon find out.

Gaps in memory

My story seems seamless as I retell it, but let me assure you it wasn't. It was full of holes and memory gaps. Sometimes when there were big chunks of time I couldn't recall, Susan would tell me stories to jog my memory, like the stories of Loretta and Tony you will soon be reading. Other times Susan called my wife Jesse to see what she remembered. Fortunately she remembered a whole lot more than I did. Codreamers frequently know our story better than we do! They're outside looking in while we're inside struggling.

Here's why you need others to codream with you

"Remember, the holographic brain and Dr. Pribram's statement, 'The more detail your hologram has, the more power it has.'

When other people hold the details of your hologram, the power of your hologram is amplified and multiplied. The more people who hold it, the more power it has. 10 people 10 times. 100 people 100 times. A million people a million times. Like computers on a network, your holographic brains are linked. Like social networks, you will be able to connect not only who *you* know but who *they* know as well, expanding your possibilities of finding support and expertise," added Susan.

SUCCESS FILE

Time to Success File again
Diet Skill Five: Switching…turning negatives into positives and forward movement

What negatives have you noticed yourself thinking or saying? I can't, I never, it's impossible to, I'll never... Whoa! Stop.

Do you have old memories associated with these doubts? What do you want to experience instead? Take a minute to switch them into positives.

How would you like the situation to turn out this time? Program a powerful new hologram in your Razz *so it can guide you past your past to your desired future.*

For the next 24 hours, pay close attention to your negative thoughts and consciously switch them as soon as they appear. Remember, what you think is what you get, like it or not.

When have you succeeded in switching someone else? You are probably great at switching your kids and friends when they're stuck in negative! Now it's time to begin switching your thoughts before your brain begins creating what you don't want!

It's time to see you successful at losing weight and gaining health. Successful at switching your old life into the one you dream!

Turn to the back of the book now and add as many more Successes as you can.

Diet Skill Six: Codreaming or co-dreading... the difference between fat and slim

"Once you have a detailed hologram in mind, the next step is to transmit your details into other people's holographic brains so you can find codreamers. To codream, they will need to be able to see what you see, hear what you hear, feel, taste and even smell what you smell. Sharing holographic details is the essence of communication... successful communication!

Codreamers are people who hold the details of your dream with you and help energize your dream. They may even hold and energize it *for you* when the going gets tough and you move into fear or doubt. Your codreamer may be a spouse or life partner, a childhood friend or someone you just happen to meet as you pursue your new lifestyle.

How can you help someone become a codreamer? Bottom line, you let them preview *the movie* of your new life... your slim, trim body, what you will look like, how you will feel, and how positively different your life will be.

If they can imagine you starring in *your movie*, if it matches their sense of your needs and abilities, as well as their ideas and beliefs, they will be able to hold your dream until you can complete it. And even believe when you get caught in doubt and resistance.

When we make changes in our lives, we need codreamers, people who travel the path with us and encourage us along the way. Let me tell you about a couple who were powerful codreamers."

Are you supersizing your body too?

Loretta was heading into one of Atlanta's high-end, glass-fronted commercial properties with a client when she saw a huge woman in the window. With a shudder she realized, "Oh my God, that's me!

I finally got it. I'm huge!"

How did this happen to me? Loretta wondered

Loretta's father was a lawyer in Southeast Asia when she was young so she grew up eating the small portions of fish and meat and generous servings of fresh vegetables and fruit that are traditional in that area. Weight was never a problem for her or her family.

Unlike the woman Loretta saw reflected in that window, she had always been an athlete. She was a state champion in backstroke as a girl, and a first team All America soccer and lacrosse player in high school and college. She was active and outdoorsy.

75 pounds... the hidden inconvenience of convenience foods!

But at 40, Loretta stopped eating and exercising the way she had all her life and slid into a life of stress and inactivity. Loretta was literally working 70 hours a week to develop her career. Real estate was her life. She woke at 5:30 am and worked till 1 am. She knew anything and everything there was to know. She was at the top of her game.

And her boyfriend John was at the top of his game too. He had just retired from the Navy, bought a sailboat and was conducting charter trips. A great life that also took about 70 hours a week so they spent evenings together.

They fell in love, got married, bought a house... and started eating together.

Bad food choices and a whole lot of denial. Does that sound familiar?

Work would keep them busy until seven or eight at night, they'd have a cocktail or two to unwind. Suddenly they'd realize it was 10 pm. "Forget cooking, let's order in"... Chinese, pizza, hi carb, hi fat and high salt. The newly-weds had a "big ole party for a couple of years." John became not just her partner in life but her partner in their *weight-gaining crime*.

One day Loretta woke up "obese and unhappy, puffy and feeling like crap." She was wearing her husband's pants and Hawaiian shirts, because none of her clothes fit. "Bad food choices and a whole lot of denial. I really didn't think I was that big until I saw myself in that window. What a wake-up call that was!"

The foods Loretta was eating were different than the ones she had eaten growing up, but the foods John was eating were pretty much the same ones he had at home. John's family was poor. They had to buy potatoes and pasta just to fill everybody up. John would never think of making a great big salad with leafy greens, fresh tomatoes, peppers and cucumbers." If I make it, he'll eat it but, left to his own devices, he will eat carbs."

Loretta finally decided to lose weight and she tried every diet under the sun... Atkins, liquid, Jenny Craig, Nutrisystem, The Cookie Diet (she said her hair fell out when she was on that one), The Grapefruit Diet and probably a couple of others she's now forgotten. She would lose 20 pounds and gain them all back. She yo yo'd up and down until she became so discouraged that she quit.

She had been dieting alone and John was continuing to eat his same old way. Their lifestyle wasn't working, and Loretta had to decide. Would she make a life-altering change, with or without

John? Or would she accept the weight she was now? But the weight she was now was unacceptable to her. She looked and felt awful.

Loretta and John decided to do Weight Watchers together

In a major sit down, Loretta and John made a pact. Instead of Loretta trying to diet alone, they decided to go to Weight Watchers together. The first month Loretta lost 14 pounds and John lost 20! The Weight Watchers' point system worked well for them. It taught them to be conscious about everything they ate and it gave them added points when they increased their exercise. Instead of eating *unconsciously*, they learned to eat *consciously*. They were both using the same plan and eating the same foods which made dieting far easier.

The first 35 pounds came off fast. In just 3 months Loretta slimmed down from 225 to 190. She had a lot more energy and felt better too, but when she looks back now, she can see she was still huge. For the next 6 months, she stayed at 190 pounds. Then Loretta decided to increase her exercise.

Until then, losing weight had been more about looking and feeling good than about health, but all that changed with one phone call. Loretta's brother was diagnosed with stage four Lung Cancer. "This knocked some sense into us. What are we doing? Throwing our lives away?" Together Loretta and John worked even harder at losing weight and exercising.

The first year Loretta's brother fought his cancer and seemed to be improving. "John and I gained amazing strength from his struggle, but within 2 years he was dead at 46. After my brother died, I cried the last 40 pounds off."

More obstacles were on the way for these committed Codreamers

Several months before, Loretta had torn her rotator cuff playing tennis. She was healing well until the weekend they returned home from her brother's funeral. She was walking their big chocolate Lab Hershey on a retractable leash. Hershey saw a squirrel and ran after it, literally shredding what was left of Loretta's partially-healed rotator cuff.

Loretta worked to rehab her shoulder until the rehab told her it's getting worse not better. You need surgery. So Loretta went to Dr. Kaplan, head of sports medicine at the University of Miami, who said her injury was worse than some Dolphin's players' injuries he works on! He didn't know how Loretta and her Lab had done so much damage.

Loretta's surgery really sidelined her. She had been walking, running and biking but now she was in a cast with her shoulder immobilized for six weeks. Having battled her way this far, this latest setback was depressing.

Loretta was thankful to have John as her codreamer. "At first he had to push me hard. I was heavily medicated and not myself. I could have let this pain take me back to Chinese food and pizza, but I didn't." A few days later, instead of wallowing in self pity, with John's help she rolled out of bed and started walking again. Her first walk was 5 miles, which was a little too ambitious. Even though she was still in pain, she walked, added distance and kept walking. Then she walked, added squats and lunges, and kept walking. Loretta must have looked strange to her neighbors she recalls, but she didn't care what anyone thought as long as she and John knew she was improving.

Committing to losing weight and supporting each other made their marriage stronger. Now Loretta's brother's death was making them rethink their lives and values even more deeply.

Loretta's brother worked hard to provide for his family, to be an honorable man and do all the right things so for him to be dealt that deck of cards, and die at 46, just didn't seem fair. "His death forever changed how I feel about my life commitments," Loretta said. "Yes, I still like making a good living. But being healthy and happy is what it's all about for me."

John and Loretta changed but John's family continued in their old poor-diet direction. Today 50% of them are at least 100 pounds overweight.

At 18, his cousin already weighs 290 pounds. Each of his parents weighs over 300. His Mom knew she needed help when she started baking and icing a cake for dinner in the morning, eating it all during the day and then having to bake and ice a second cake so no one would find out. Five years ago, she had Lap Band surgery and regained all her weight. Now she's back to drinking two to three large bottles of Coke a day, eating a half dozen eggs, half a loaf of bread and two pieces of apple pie with ice cream for breakfast! Yes, you read that right... for breakfast. For dinner, she downs two whole chickens with mac and cheese, or a mound of frozen chicken tenders and lots of potatoes.

Three out of four of John's cousins are at least 100 pounds overweight. The 4th cousin has gone all the way over to the other side. Bravo! She gets up at 3 am every day to walk and she is the only one who is keeping her weight stable. His younger brother is 200 plus pounds overweight. John's three obese cousins are in their 40s and 50s and major health issues are cropping up... diabetes, high blood pressure, back pain and immobility. One cousin can't walk or work and is on permanent disability. All of their children are at least 100 pounds overweight... severely obese.

John's family has made poor food choices generation after generation. Sadly, somebody was putting junk food in front of them as children and it's affecting their whole lives. *Unfortunately this family is just one example of a big slice of the American pie.*

Not everyone is as fortunate as Loretta. Not everyone has family support. But most of us do have a friend!

Highly-valued codreamers

Yes, it's important to hear other people's success stories, not just as brief conversational summaries but stories told in depth. Understanding their process helps us become more aware of our own. I have been fortunate to have many codreamers in my life, my wife, my congregants, my friends.

Stacey can plant far-bigger holograms, or in this case far-smaller holograms, in Jesse's mind than Jesse can herself. One day when they were walking behind a trim 19-year-old wearing skin-tight white pants outside Miami Juice, Jesse exclaimed, See that's why I can never wear white pants. You have to look like THAT to wear them! Stacey exclaimed back even louder and more firmly, "Yes you can wear white pants. And I can already see you looking great in them!"

Today Jesse is still holding Stacey's hologram. She visualizes herself looking great in white pants, maybe not as slim as that 19-year-old but just as good in her own way! Now Jesse is codreaming with Stacey. And she's just about ready to go buy those white pants.

My wife Jesse is a powerful codreamer and shield. I've always known that, even though I didn't have these words to describe it. But I never realized that choosing Jesse as my wife and codreamer was actually a success skill. Now, Susan, I can see clearly that it was.

I have friends who have gone on diet after diet and their spouses and family members, despite numerous requests, have continued to bring home tempting foods, put cookies in the cabinets and ice cream in the freezer, which sooner or later they succumbed to and consumed. Or, family members who were constantly filled with doubts and discouraging comments, put-downs and jeers like, Why don't you just give up! Enough is enough.

Thank you, Jesse, from the bottom of my heart. I am most blessed to have you as my wife, my codreamer and shield. And thank you, Susan, for making me aware.

The difference between success and failure, between health and obesity frequently boils down to two simple questions: Do you have codreamers? And do you have the expertise and knowledge you need?

The restaurant owner didn't greet me

Here is a story that made me feel very acknowledged for my weight loss. I went to a restaurant I hadn't been to for a while. It's one I have been going to since it opened. The owner, a local celebrity from Uruguay and family friend, is always in the dining room greeting guests. But this evening he failed to greet me with his usual bear hug.

I wondered if it was because we hadn't been splurging on various steak specialties and racking up huge bills. We used to order a steak for each person at the table and the owner would always send over a waiter to prepare their famous flaming dessert... caramel filled crepes doused with brandy, set ablaze and topped with vanilla ice cream.

Instead of making up reasons why he had not greeted me, I stood up and headed toward him with both arms open wide, Hello my friend, did I do something wrong? With a sparkle in his eye, he laughed and opened his arms too.

"Oh, is that you, Rabbi? I didn't recognize you. What did you do? You look so much younger." Yes, my friend," I replied. I have changed my ways and my body. You also look much younger and fitter. Even though my food needs have changed, I still want to eat here so please share a few secrets from your kitchen with me.

Which items on your menu fit my new healthier lifestyle? What do you eat from this menu? He told me that he could prepare lots of delicious dishes for me. His favorite grilled chicken is flavored with simple herbs, garlic and lemon. His meats are broiled without any added fat and the fat drains away during cooking. His vegetables are roasted on an open fire with no added salt.

Somewhere in that conversation, we became codreamers. Now whenever Jesse and I eat in his restaurant, he excitedly tells my weight-loss story to everyone who is there. He's part of my team and getting others interested in eating our new way too.

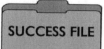

SUCCESS FILE

Time to Success File again
Diet Skill Six: Codreaming to find the support you need

Who are your codreamers? That is, who are the people who hold the details of your dreams with you? Who do you share your tiny forward steps with, bounce your ideas around with, and celebrate your successes with?

Do you have a lot of codreamers or only one or two? Who else would you like to have codream with you? Who else do you plan to share the details of your new holographic dreams with? Remember, the more detail, the more power. And the more codreamers you have, the more your dream's power is multiplied.

Who have you discovered is a co-dreader not a codreamer? Maybe that discovery comes as a shock to you. But knowing that now can be very valuable to you in the future!

Who are you codreaming with? Who has entrusted his or her precious dream with you? Are you up-to-date with his or her latest details? Have you Success Filed with him or her lately?

Which of your codreamers is good at switching you? Is it time to call your codreamers and codream your next level?

Turn to the back of the book now and add as many more successes as you can to your Success File.

Diet Skill Seven: Finding experts... who are also codreamers

For millions of people, Weight Watchers, Jenny Craig, Biggest Loser, Slim-Fast, Flat Belly, Nutrisystem, Abs Diet, South Beach, The Zone and other diet programs provide the expertise and structure they need to lose weight in 1st gear. Most diets work well short term, for a few weeks or months. But then the real question presents itself. Do you have the success skills and expertise to lose weight *not just short term but long term as well*?

Weight Watchers worked well for Loretta and John, especially since they had a powerful additional *success ingredient... they were codreamers.* They did it together, in good times and bad, and together they are now celebrating the joys of their new health.

Maybe your expert is a personal trainer or a nutritionist. An expert in sports medicine, a chiropractor or acupuncturist. A group fitness instructor at the Y or in your neighborhood, or the coach of a team you have joined. Remember this, your expert's credentials, licenses and references are a good start but they don't tell the whole story!

Beware, not all experts want what you want!
"Some experts will try to overwhelm your hologram and insert the details of their hologram in your head and emotions. *Just because someone is an expert doesn't mean he or she will be willing, or able, to codream with you.*

Have you ever hired a designer or architect who tried to talk you out of what you really wanted, and you bought it? Or a computer or TV salesman? A car salesman or friend? A makeup artist or hair stylist? It's up to you to find experts who will codream with you.

Your expert needs to have the heart of a teacher and the skills of a leader, not just the mind of a profit-driven business person.

Experts 101... more than anyone ever taught you

Let's take a few minutes to update what you know about finding and using experts. As you search for an expert, keep the three gears of success in mind. Which gear are you in this area? Are you a beginner? Do you already have some skills and experience? Or are you creating something brand new, a new design, a new product or service? Are you in 1st Gear, 2nd or 3rd? Or are you shifting from one gear to another? **Remember you *and your expert* need to operate in the right gear at the right time**.

Some experts get stuck... will you get stuck with them!

To find the right expert at the right time, you need to become skillful at giving and receiving word cues. Let's take a minute to review your gear-shifting word cues...

If you hear these words, you know this person is operating in first gear: right/wrong, good/bad, should/shouldn't, have to/must, always/never, safe/dangerous, correct/incorrect, scared, worried, doubtful, nervous, hesitant, anxious, frightened, fearful, trying, pleasing, obedient and loyal.

Listen to the words you are using as well. Do your word cues and theirs match? Are you operating in the same gear at the same time?

When you or your teacher shifts into 2nd gear, you will hear a whole new set of word signals: more-better-faster, more repetitions, more stretch and extension, more exertion, more flexibility, more sweat, more strength, more endurance, better/worse, longer/harder, quantity/quality, competition, scores, charts, prizes, stress, burnout and injuries.

When you have shifted into 3rd gear you and your expert will be using new words: create, realize, how about, what if, I have an idea, here's a possibility, what do you think, let's look at this, Aha!, cooperation, communication, teamwork, mission, balance, integrity, choice and ease.

Is your expert able to operate in all three gears along with you? Or do your gears grind and screech? Do you feel your expert is pulling you in another direction and forcing you to bend and yield? Is your expert available, as available as you need her or him to be?

Vet the input you get. A lesson Dylan had to learn

Is your expert an authority, or an authority figure? Someone the-child-in-you was taught to respect, someone "older and wiser" but not necessarily someone who is an expert in this area.

For years, my grandson Dylan thought I knew everything! But then he began to see that there are limits to what I know. And he had to begin asking himself, is Mama (the name he chose for me when he first began to talk) the best person to ask about this topic, or do I need to find a new authority? An expert in that field?

Who do you listen to? And whose authority-figure status could send you *off course*? Whose disagreement might overwhelm you? Whose well-defined, highly-detailed holograms might you unconsciously substitute for yours, and regret later?

My mom said, my dad said, my lawyer told me, I heard it on TV or I read it on the internet. Vet the input you receive so you can stay on course. Whose critique should you pay attention to? And whose should you ignore... or take with a grain of salt!

Take a good hard look at your experts too. If they are not living the lifestyle you have in mind, if they are not healthy, fit and in shape, you may need to rethink how closely you follow their advice.

Machete experts... cut, cut, chop, chop

Here's a key question. Does your potential expert align with the details of your dream or desired outcome? Or does he or she go at it with axes and machetes and chop it apart? Do you feel dazed and disoriented after sharing it? Is what's left of your dream still attractive to you? Or does it feel like the dream of an alien from Mars's, but definitely not yours?

Like a gardener tending a tiny plant, can your expert nurture your tender, young dream so it can grow and thrive? Can he or she codream and co-create it with you?

Ok, you've found an expert. But is he or she a good teacher?

Next, you need to discover whether your potential expert/codreamer is also a good teacher. Someone who remembers what it was like to be in 1st gear... the constant attention you need, the simple, precise directions you want to be given. The million and one questions you want answers to. How else are you going to learn?

In 1st gear, your experts need to listen, really listen... and make your goals their goals. They need to sense when you need more control and when you need more freedom. They need to be supportive when you need support and tough when you need toughness. Your expert needs to believe in your ability to succeed and when the limits of how far he or she can take you, be willing and able to pass you on to other experts who can take you to your next level.

Most important of all in 1st gear, your expert will need to remember how important it is for you to feel success-full each day. He or she needs to help you add as many new successes to your Success File as possible.

Fortunately you don't have to become an expert in all areas. You can find trained, skillful experts to assist you... a personal trainer, a nutritionist, a physician or weight loss program, a personal shopper or stylist... people who can help you build a hologram that is bigger and bolder than you can even dare imagine alone!" smiled Susan.

Best exercise tips I've ever gotten were given free by someone beside me

Ask questions. Be a keen observer. Make friends. Some of the best advice I've ever gotten was given to me by someone who was working out next to me.

If you can afford to hire a trainer, fine, but you don't have to hire a $100 an hour trainer at this point. You can take a class at the Y or your gym, join a team or practice with a DVD an expert has created.

Success has 3 gears and so does leadership

"Remember the 3 gears of success. Well, there are also 3 gears of leadership. You will want to understand each one thoroughly before you invest time and money in experts... teachers, trainers and coaches because they probably won't be aware of which leadership gears use.

There are experts who can only operate in one gear. And there are experts who can shift up and down in all three gears as needed. *Unfortunately* most experts don't know which leadership gears they are using. So you will have to figure that out for yourself!

Here's how to recognize which gear of leadership you need. 1st gear experts can tell you how to do it correctly and safely. 2nd gear experts can show you how to do it more-better-faster. They're skilled and experienced. And 3rd gear experts can help you design and create holograms and bring them into reality. There are some experts who only use one gear and there are others you use all three. They are Three-Gear Leaders," explained Susan.

TV experts are powerful codreamers

Trainers on *The Biggest Loser* and *Extreme Makeover: Weight Loss Edition* are powerful experts and codreamers. These shows are valuable and inspiring to watch. They let you experience the process weight-losers go through day-by-day, step by step. They will help you clarify your vision and show you how to manage plateaus and setbacks. And these shows also let you experience what powerful, codreamer/experts are like.

When you reach out for experts keep this story in mind. As you read it, think about what you want and need from experts as you lose weight, increase exercise and gain health.

If Tony can do it, you can do it too

What's possible? Seems like a complicated question, but it's not.

What's possible to our brains is what's already been done. What hasn't been done is temporarily impossible. Here is a story that may make your impossible possible.

He wanted to lose 200 pounds by his 50th birthday

Tony, a 49 year old hardworking pizza restaurant manager, hadn't weighed himself for two years because he couldn't find scale strong enough, even at his doctor's. When he was chosen to participate on Extreme Makeover: Weight Loss Edition, his trainer Chris Powell took him to the freight scale at a truck loading dock and Tony weighed in at a whopping 398 pounds!

The image of a man being weighed on a freight scale overwhelmed Tony and he sobbed in embarrassment, but he used that embarrassment to give himself a life-changing gift. He committed to weigh an even 200 pounds, to be "sexy and slim" on his 50th birthday in one year.

23 gallons of fat! He drank 2,000 calories a day... before eating anything

Tony went through a battery of tests and his doctor told him he was literally carrying around *23 gallons of fat*. Yes, think about that for a minute. His arms and legs were normal in size, but the excess weight he was carrying was all around his middle. This fat, belly fat and visceral fat, is associated with a higher risk of heart attack. His doctor said Tony was lucky. People as overweight as you are usually dead by age 50. Tony was in danger of leaving his sons without a father. And, almost as upsetting, of always having his sons remember him as fat. Not an example he wanted to set.

With spousal support, your success rate is 4 times higher

Tony's weight loss plan was divided into four 90 day phases and weigh-ins.

For someone carrying an extra 200 pounds, the daily workouts were grueling. Tony kept smiling and pressing himself and Chris kept smiling and pressing Tony too... weight training three days a week and cardio six days. A new body was what Tony wanted for his birthday and he was determined to do whatever it took.

*Extreme Make*over renovated the home Tony and his fiancée were sharing, added a new kitchen, new bedrooms, a new living room and state-of-the-art work out equipment. His trainer Chris moved in with them to be there for Tony 24/7 during those critical first three months. Tony's goal was to lose 100 pounds while Chris was there coaching him. While he was in 1st gear.

Chris introduced Tony to a nutritionist who taught him how to cook in new healthy ways, grilling chicken and making fish tacos that were tasty and delicious as well as low-calorie and low-fat. She explained to Tony that he had been *consuming 2,000 or more calories a day just in the large cups of juice he drank with his meals...* 2,000 calories it would take 8 hours in the gym to work off. She suggested Tony drink no-sugar green tea with a non-nutrient sweetener instead.

The Holiday Trap... pies, cakes, cookies and breads

During the first three months Tony was doing well, but his fiancée and potential codreamer was not. She could have participated and lost weight herself, instead she saw Tony's commitment to his food and exercise plan as taking him away from her. She nagged and complained especially on Christmas when she

128

wanted Tony to eat all the pies, cakes, cookies and breads everyone else was eating, but he stuck to his plan.

We can empathize with Tony and Leslie. Christmas... pies, cakes, cookies and breads Mom made and the family had enjoyed traditionally. Celebration holograms which have been made more and more highly detailed and powerful over the years compete with newer less familiar, less powerful holograms. Tony had to put forth a gigantic act of will to complete his Christmas day food plan *without Leslie's support.*

When you were stressed, upset, worried, disappointed, sad and depressed, what comfort foods did you eat? Sweet, salty, alcoholic, cold or hot? How else can you deal with these negative emotions? It is time to create new stress-reducing holograms that will empower you to lose weight and gain health, no matter what or when. And to pre-experience living them over and over to make them powerful and familiar.

Life doesn't stop throwing obstacles your way just because you're on a diet

While Tony was working out, his phone rang. His son Marcus, who had been born with cerebral palsy and miraculously survived past childhood, was in critical condition in another city. Tony's ex-wife said there was nothing he could do for Marcus. Marcus would want you to stay and fight for your life too. She promised to stay in touch.

Chris saw Tony's weight-loss results slowing down. Chris tried to help Tony's fiancée get on board and she kept saying, "I want to." Finally Chris retorted firmly, "But will you?" Leslie didn't, and her negative reactions continued. Tony was forced to choose between his commitment to life, and his commitment to marrying Leslie. He chose life! The engagement was off and Tony moved out of their shared home.

Success Filing Tony's first three months

Tony's most thrilling early successes included: My pants fell down around my ankles. My clothes were too big... freakin' amazing! I had to punch holes in my belt and put on suspenders to hold up my pants. And, "Chris, for the first time in my life, I don't have to turn to food. I turn to exercise. I learned that from you."

At his three month weigh-in, Tony was down from 398 to 294

Despite all his challenges, at three months, *Tony made his 100 pound weight-loss goal plus an additional four pounds*. His weight was down from 398 to 294.

The other side of Tony's success... a powerful 1st gear expert/codreamer

Chris Powell is well known for working with the extremely obese. He understood the pressures of 1st gear so well that he arranged to live with Tony during those crucial first 90 days... the days when Tony didn't know what to do, when he could injure himself if he exercised incorrectly. The times when past experiences and old habits would press hardest against him, when other people in his life could get in the way, when he most needed his expert beside him, to correct and acknowledge him, to build his skills and self-confidence.

Chris knew what it would take for Tony to lose 200 pounds and he guided him there step-by-step, from the first weigh-in, medical workup and OK. From the early "flight or fight workout" when Chris tested Tony's commitment by pushing him way beyond his limits and pointing to the door. But no door for Tony. He got back on the treadmill and kept going.

Your success gear and your leader's gear must match

Chris led Tony in whichever gear he needed. When Tony was in 1st gear, Chris was in the 1st gear of leadership, motivating and encouraging him. He made sure Tony learned basic food and exercise skills. He was caring but tough. He acknowledged his successes and corrected his failures, nurturing and motivating him each step of the way, even promising Tony and Leslie their dream honeymoon when Tony lost his first 100 pounds.

At the end of three months when Tony was ready to shift into 2nd gear independence, Chris geared up into 2nd gear leadership and moved out as planned. Under normal circumstances, Tony would have easily met his next goal. He had the skills, he had a full Success File and he was committed to his outcome.

But nothing was normal for Tony after that

Tony was in 2nd gear in his diet and exercise program, but when his engagement ended and Chris moved out as planned, even though Tony told Chris he had a place to live, Tony unexpectedly found himself in 1st gear in the rest of his life... with no bed to sleep in, no kitchen to cook in and no regular place to exercise. Tony didn't want to go back to managing a pizza restaurant, the lifestyle that made him fat. He planned to start his own security business, but getting started was tougher than he thought and he ran out of money.

Before Chris left, he repeatedly told Tony to call him whenever he had problems or questions and Tony promised to do that, but Tony didn't call. Back in California, Chris had no way of knowing that Tony was homeless, living in his car, exercising in parks and up and down stairwells. Despite repeated efforts, Chris was unable to locate him until finally the show's producer spotted Tony's car, loaded with all his possessions, in a parking garage the day before his next weigh in.

Reaching out for help is essential in 2nd gear

In 2nd gear when your expert is no longer beside you to see how you are doing, reaching out to ask for help is an essential skill. Tony let his pride prevent him from getting the support he needed. He had basic needs that were unmet… the need to have a new job so he could earn money, the need to have a home and bed so he could eat, rest and feel safe. Tony didn't tell anyone in his family he was homeless either. If he had, one of them might have reached out to Chris on Tony's behalf.

Not reaching out for help took its toll

At his six-month weigh-in, Tony failed to come even close to his goal. In fact he missed it by 50%. That meant at the end of the next three months, Tony would not only have to lose the weight he agreed on but he would also have to lose the weight failed to lose. A tough assignment because success at the nine-month weigh-in was crucial.

Tony would be meeting with a surgeon to determine whether or not he was a candidate for skin-removing surgery… a highly-motivating bonus. Tony had huge masses of flesh hanging from his belly and thighs. "I want to be able to look down and *see my own toes!*"

In 2nd gear, Chris helped Tony meet his unmet 1st gear needs

Does your expert have the skills to lead you in 1st gear as well as in 2nd and 3rd gears? Losing weight and exercising aren't the only things in your life. What else will your leader need to be able to help you with along the way?

Without having his 1st gear needs met, Chris knew Tony would not be able to shift into 2nd gear so his codreamer/expert Chris stepped in to help. He offered to let Tony come and stay in his home, but Tony was starting his business so he needed to stay put. Understanding Tony's needs better, Chris offered to send Tony to a training program to be certified as a personal guard so he could begin earning money. This time Tony set his pride aside and accepted help, and his weight loss dream was revitalized.

Tony was a man on fire. At his 9 month weigh-in, Tony had lost 172 pounds and weighed 226! And his medical tests were so good that he qualified for skin-removing surgery with flying colors. Tony was elated.

From the heights to the depths

Tony received another devastating call. His son Marcus was dead, yet another moment when other people might have given up. But with Chris's guidance, Tony valiantly pursued his weight loss goals in his son's memory. Marcus became his inspiration and determination.

A country of codreamers celebrated Tony's 50th birthday

The day of Tony's weigh-in was a day of great celebration. *Extreme Makeover* introduced Tony to a whole country of codreamers. People everywhere watched and cheered Tony on, and a whole country of codreamers were proud when Tony stepped out of an SUV onto the beach looking "sexy and slim."

Tony had lost 200 pounds in a year

Tony weighed in amidst anticipatory silence and, yes, from 398 to 198, Tony had lost 200 pounds in one year! And he received once again the gift God had given him at birth... the gift of a slim, fit, healthy Miraculous Body.

A month later, Tony dropped to his knee and proposed, not to his old fiancée, but to Deanna, a beautiful new codreamer Tony met along the way.

Together or apart, Chris held Tony's dream

Chris was constantly there with Tony in those first three grueling months. He worried when he saw Tony's relationship with Leslie coming apart and helped him move out when it was clear the engagement was over. When Marcus died, Chris surprised Tony by flying across the country to stand beside him and his family at the funeral.

Tony's success was not just because Chris was an expert. Even more important, Chris was a codreamer who beamed ear-to-ear when Tony stepped out on his 50th birthday looking "sexy and slim" at 198 pounds. Half the man he used to be and twice the person.

When you are a codreamer, your partner's success is your success too, your success as a leader like Chris.

Tony's story brought a flood of memories!

I have been fortunate to have a powerful 3rd gear expert and codreamer in my life. Like Chris, Larry has been there for me each step of the way.

Larry is a world-class physician, dermatologist and internist

Larry is older than I am but just as spirited and inquisitive. He was educated at the Citadel, served in the military and received his medical training at the University of Georgia. Despite fighting battles with his health, he has remained fit and energetic all his life. And he needs to be fit to serve his 40,000-patient practice. For me, one of Larry's best qualities is that he is successful in business but never greedy in life.

Larry and his wife Sandy have been my great supporters. Not only do they believe I can succeed in my weight-loss challenges, but they also support me with any other challenges I face. Larry has always been available to give medical input or to help me understand the changes that were going on in my body whether I hit a plateau or wasn't getting enough sleep. He let me know when I was on the right track and when I wasn't, and all the latest studies to show to my doctor.

I tend to push too hard so Larry is there to tell me when I need to slow down, when I need to update and make changes. When I have a certain pain, he tells me which exercise to do instead. He gives me guidelines, do's and don'ts like never use public yoga mats or public Jacuzzis. When I damaged my rotator cuff, I consulted with Larry before and after my workouts to make sure I did not damage it further.

Often when we call each other, we discuss health. One of the topics we address is percentage of body fat. Although Larry supports me in my weight loss goals, he also wants to make sure I maintain a healthy level of body fat. Larry reminds me that normal fat storage is 12% in men and 15% in women. This quantity of fat is needed for metabolism and to ensure proper function. He reminds me to maintain adequate hydration and electrolytes. Recently we have been talking about wheat and gluten and how they slow down weight loss.

Larry is a congregant of our synagogue and he is also my best friend and most trusted doctor. As a dermatologist, he has always taught me that re-establishing a person's self confidence is as important as restoring that person's health.

Pay half price because he's only getting half a rabbi

Larry likes to joke that Rabbi Cukierkorn has lost so much weight that "I should only have to pay half the synagogue dues because I'm only getting half a Rabbi!"

Like Tony, Larry lost his son

Larry has dealt with adversities few people have to face, but he has dealt with those tragedies and setbacks in a very functional, compassionate and successful way. I only hope that I will have the grace to do the same.

As a rabbi, I am called to be there for people in very painful times. And this was one call that made me dig deep.

I buried Larry's son

David was a bright, handsome, athletic 27-year-old restaurant owner. The day before he was killed by a hit and run driver, he closed his restaurant at noon to go buy bicycles and deliver them to a group foster home.

Larry's son David also bought Christmas toys for children he didn't know, to celebrate a holiday he didn't celebrate himself. That's just how generous and sensitive he was. David had made so many friends that when I conducted his funeral, there were over a 1,000 people there. The police had to close the main road and direct traffic so hundreds of others who just wanted to offer condolences to his family could get in.

Staring at the picture of David his family had on display at the funeral made me feel that his death was an even greater loss. He was living his life to the fullest and helping others live their lives to the fullest too. Ironically David Hudson was killed by another David who had racked up several DUIs and was on a very different path. People make very different choices in life.

Even though David Hudson is dead, I always remember him alive and vital, giving the way he did that last day at a group foster home. When I die, I hope to be remembered as having lived a life worth living and having the kind of vitality and generosity David had. Larry's son David continues to be a source of inspiration for me, and I hope he will be for you too.

A time I should have reached out for expertise, but I didn't

I could relate to Tony when he was homeless and he didn't call Chris to let him know he needed help. I didn't reach out to Larry at a time when I should have.

On a plane trip from Mexico City to Veracruz, I sat next to a very heavy man wearing denim overalls. I speak Spanish so we started talking. He told me he was a physician who had a practice in

Juarez and his entire business was prescribing diet meds for people in America. Could you tell me which medicines you prescribe for people? That's easy, I just prescribe one. Subitramine. Would you please write that name down for me and the number of milligrams I should take? He told me to take one 15 mg pill each morning.

How much do I owe you? No, I like you Rabbi. And he asked me for a blessing.

When I arrived in Veracruz, as I was walking down the street I saw a pharmacy and went in. I showed the woman the handwritten note he had scribbled on my In Flight magazine. In Mexico, I guess that was enough to be a prescription. They said they didn't have 15 mg they only had 30. Can I cut them in half? No, they are capsules. But people take 30 mg all the time and they're the same price. So I figured I could lose twice as much weight for half the price.

I planned to get home and research the product before I took it, but when I realized Subitramine was the same as Meridia which was FDA approved for weight loss in the U.S., I decided to start taking it without checking into it further.

The first day on the drug, I was so sped up that I literally ran up and down the halls and stairwells of our building. I really wanted to call Larry because for the last 5 years I hadn't taken so much as an aspirin without consulting him, but I was embarrassed that I had purchased diet medicine without a prescription from "a drugstore" in Mexico. And had taken it.

Within a week, I could see how well the drug suppressed my appetite and I was losing weight. I took the drug for four months and lost 18 pounds but I began to notice that my heart seemed to be racing all the time and I heard on TV that the FDA was considering pulling Meridia off the market. Three million prescriptions had been filled in the U.S. by that time. But the FDA didn't pull Meridia and simply kept a watch on it.

Finally in 2010, Abbott Laboratories took Meridia off the market, "citing evidence that Meridia was associated with 84 deaths, 11 of which were people who were under 30 years old, and thousands of reactions such as rapid heart rate, high blood pressure, and heart palpitations." I realized that no matter what the FDA said or did, I should have been paying more attention to my own body. The FDA was waiting for more deaths and I didn't want to be one of them.[21]

In one of my conversations with Larry, I finally said I had something I needed to tell him. The truth is I have been on Meridia for 4 months. I'm scared to tell you but I'm more scared not to. But because Larry has been a doctor much longer than he's been my friend, there was no judgment. He simply told me, "I want you to stop taking that drug right now."

Larry recommended that my doctor do a full round of exams to make sure my heart had not been compromised. Fortunately my heart was fine.

It was a disappointing experience, but the person I was most disappointed in was me. I had gone with the advice of someone who did not have my best interests at heart. It was an expensive mistake, but the upside was that I was scared into taking better care of myself, and being far more careful about the products I consume.[22]

Sometimes it's tough to be a codreamer

Codreamers are emotionally engaged in your Dream. They go through your ups and downs with you. They hold on when you seem to be going off the rails. And they hold you when you are about to let go.

For my codreamer wife Jesse, those were scary days. She had been frightened when I started taking Meridia. She saw how sped up I was, even though at first I was enjoying having so much energy. She worried that her husband hadn't known enough about that doctor and hadn't reached out to Larry to ask about Meridia before he started taking it. She had also urged me to call Larry and was happy when I finally did.

Like Tony, I had to overcome my embarrassment and pride. It wasn't like me to do such a careless thing. And, given how much I dislike blood tests and procedures, it was a hard lesson for us both.

For Jesse there is also a very bright side to being my codreamer. Jesse's vision of our future together has changed drastically during the weight-loss years.

Jesse no longer pictures her husband growing old like his father, spending more and more time in bed in pain and eating all his meals there during his later years.

Jesse has a new view, "I visualize us traveling, hiking up mountains, participating in a triathlon together. I can picture us having the energy to swim with our grandchildren, after enjoying Sophie's wedding of course. Or going for long walks on the beach and looking cute in our jeans as we grow older."

Experts may be good at what they do, but do they feel good *to you*?

When you choose experts, check their credentials and recommendations *but also be sure to* check out *how they feel to you*. The real question isn't just... Are they good at what they do? It's also, Are they good for you? Can they give you feedback in a positive, supportive way, a way that motivates and inspires you? *Even though it's tough love, you should still know it's love.*

Your expert may advise and inform you. Your expert may motivate and challenge you, *but if you consistently feel contradicted or opposed, find someone else to be your expert.* Yes, YOUR expert. An expert who is also YOUR codreamer.

Pain is a great teacher if you learn from it. And Dmitry did

At 25 Dmitry looked terrific. He was a handsome, blond, young man from freezing cold Siberia who moved to steaming hot Miami to work in the cruise industry. He looked healthy and vital, but he was in pain. Back pain. Neck pain. He couldn't sit in a car or movie for more than an hour without needing to lie down.

"My life began to nosedive. The only comfort I could find was stuffing myself with junk food. I went from eating a slice of pizza to devouring the entire pie. From ordering an omelet for breakfast to ordering a double cheeseburger, coke, fries and ice cream instead. I was caught in a trap I could not get out of. My pain was getting worse and the more I ate to comfort myself the bigger my body got. I started ordering from room service and leaving the door open so the delivery person would bring in my food and I wouldn't have to get up to open the door. I was afraid to make those extra movements because I didn't want the pain to get worse. Then I started drinking vodka until I blacked out. My weight soared from 160 to 240. I was smoking 2 packs a day. I couldn't feel my legs and I couldn't get up. Those moments scared me but instead of driving me to healthier choices they drove me to eat even more.

People around me were disgusted by how I looked and started turning away from me. A few real friends tried to help but I did not want to listen. One friend didn't recognize me because I had gotten so fat. Another friend cried when she saw me and sobbed what are you doing to yourself and your life? Dmitry, remember how you were! I reached a point when I didn't care about my life but I did care about my parents and how they would feel if they saw me. They gave me birth to me and took care of me. I realized I had to take care of myself to take care of those who loved me.

Finally a friend told Dmitry about yoga. Dmitry's response was all too familiar. I'm in too much pain to do yoga. Besides, I'm not flexible enough. But his friend cared and kept urging him. "Dmitry, you don't have to be pain-free to do yoga. Yoga will help with your pain. You don't have to be flexible to do yoga either. Yoga will help you become flexible. Just go to class and do what you can, step by step, day by day."

And Dmitry did. When he was in tremendous pain and trying to cover it up with food, it never occurred to him that exercise could be his way out. He went to yoga every day, no matter how he felt. His pain disappeared, his flexibility returned and he chose to become a certified Bikram teacher.

"I have not had pizza for so long now that I don't remember how it tastes. My weight is back down to 170 plus more muscle. Yoga changed my life. Eating healthy food, exercising, and taking care of my body and mind is my life now. I am happy where I am and happy to share my story to let people around me know that it is never too late to make a u-turn and get back on the road to health and fitness."

Dmitry became Susan' teacher

Susan wasn't in Dmitry's life during those painful years. But he came into hers when she first went to Bikram yoga… when she was in pain, when she wasn't flexible, when she was standing near the wall so she wouldn't fall on her left knee. "Dmitry and the other teachers guided me day by day, step by step until I was finally able to get in my car without even noticing I was getting in at all… the way it ought to be. Eventually I was able to sleep and turn over in the night without a half hour of sharp pain keeping me awake.

Pain is a great teacher, and someone who has skillfully moved through pain makes a great teacher. Someone like Dmitry. Or someone *like you* once you have lost weight and regained your health. As people see your body and life changing, they will begin asking you all kinds of questions. They will want to know how they can get the same result. They will ask you to be a codreamer. And maybe even a 1st gear expert, someone who will teach them the basics of a skill and the self-confidence to enjoy it."

Now Dmitry has a TV show that helps people in pain

Each week, Dmitry teaches easy yoga postures people can do whether they have arthritis or they have been immobile for a while. Susan has been a frequent guest demonstrating postures, proving that even if you are in pain and not in good shape when you start, you can help your miraculous body heal itself.

"But be aware in advance that your new lifestyle may not suit some of the people who are closest to you. In fact, it will challenge you to get clear about who is a codreamer and who isn't. From now on, you will be behaving differently, not going out so often for pizza and beer, or stopping for coffee and Danish, or spending hours indulging in rich, wine-filled dinners. Or going out with the girls and ordering martinis that taste like chocolate mint or pancakes with syrup... sugar in an elegant glass on the dessert-drink continuum.

Sad to say, some people you're close to now may decide your old lifestyle is more important than spending time with you, and they may move on. Let them. A deletion success. Others with healthy habits will soon fill their spaces, just the way Tony's new fiancée did. The new codreamers you find will probably be on a similar, healthy course. And that's good news," exclaimed Susan.

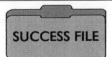

SUCCESS FILE

Time to Success File again...
Diet Skill Seven: Finding experts who are also codreamers

Which experts you know are stuck in one gear or another... perfect when you start but unable to gear up with you? Or perfect in 2nd gear but unable to gear down when you need more help, or gear up when you want creativity? And which ones are so creative they can't gear down to pass on their creative ideas and approaches, to teach others how or produce results?

Who do you turn to when you have a health issue? A food or an exercise issue? Who do you talk to when you feel you're off course or slipping into a slump? Or you think you need to update its details?

What successes have you had because you reached out to an expert? What progress did you make when you had that person's expert input and guidance? Who are the experts you regularly use? What gears are they able to operate in? And lead you in?

When did you listen to the wrong expert or not reach out at all? What did you have to do to correct that omission? How much time and energy was lost? What will do you next time!

Turn to the back of the book and add as many more Successes as you can. When your Success File is... you know the rest.

Remember, we can't do life alone.
That's why there are so many of us here on the planet!

Diet Skill Eight: Shielding... raising your infant dream

"When you birth a dream, you become responsible for its survival. You are its parent and CEO. You probably won't be able to complete it all by yourself, and you probably don't want to either. Codreamers not only amplify the power of your dream, but they are powerful shields as well.

Why do you need shields? Because there will be lots of disagreement once you proclaim your dream and start taking action, disagreement from people around you, even those closest to you," explained Susan.

Yes, I knew it. I was about to say, OK Susan, the eighth success skill is Shielding! And I remember a time when I had to shield my tender heart.

Flan, flan, flan... she wouldn't take No for an answer

My aunt makes a delicious dessert that had always been one of my favorites, flan. Flan is a thick egg custard with a caramel topping. It is made with a whole lot of sugar, is very rich and calorie-laden. My aunt had always brought flan to holiday events and dinners.

When I started my diet and we invited her to our home, she offered to bring flan and I told her I was on a diet and asked her to bring fruit. Instead she said, "OK, you are on a diet so I will bring flan for Sophie." I told her that we didn't want our daughter to have flan either because we were teaching her to make healthier food choices. But my aunt chose to bring it anyway, courting Sophie's favor but not respecting our wishes as her parents. After dinner when she served the flan, she flamboyantly insisted on offering it to me saying, *"Live a little,* eat this dessert."

And I remember responding flamboyantly, "NO, I prefer to *live a lot,* and *not* eat that dessert.

After the third time she brought flan despite our repeated requests, we decided to scale down the number of invitations we extended to her. Now when she comes to our house for dinner, she doesn't bring flan. Thank heavens that Jesse and I were aligned. I don't know whether I could have stood up to her alone!

Co-dreaders... don't let them kill your dreams!

"You will need shields to protect you from people close to you who aren't codreamers, but who are co-dreaders instead. Or just dreaders in general. There are a number of different types of shields you can use.

Codreamers can shield you from blowing off your diet or exercise or getting talked into something that will take you off course. Something like a "family member" or "a friend" who keeps offering you flan or pizza and beer or whatever foods are your favorites.

Very detailed plans and dreams are powerful shields too. Plans like knowing which foods you want to eat and which ones you want to avoid or minimize. Knowing how much sugar is in ketchup or how much sodium is in a dill pickle can be important when you're at a picnic away from home, and you're at the mercy of their menu. What else do they have on the table? Sliced tomatoes? Broccoli, cauliflower and carrots? Plain grilled chicken, sliced apples and strawberries? Knowing what you want to eat and what you want to avoid can steer you through uncertainty or persuasion, through other people's kitchens and menus.

And there are also *anticipation shields*. Yes, knowing that you are just days or weeks away from getting back into your favorite dress or slacks is another powerful shield! Or having the outfit you plan to wear to an upcoming party or dance hanging on your closet door. Yes, dance! Your desire to get into that outfit can shield you too.

There will be days...

There will be days when you will want to go off your diet with all your might. You will want to give up on your exercise plan, abandon your once-enticing dream and leave it there to shrivel up to nothing. But if you have created codreamers, they simply won't let you. "What? You can't do that. That's your dream and you've got to keep going!

They will playback the positive details you shared with them, how excited you were when you told them about your hologram and how vital it is to your health and well being. Hopefully you will have shared your Success File with them so they can remember your successes even better than you when you're in "abandon mode." What dream? I want a cookie!

Your codreamer will reload those positive details in your brain and revitalize your dream. Then, with your hologram alive and well again, you can put down that "mental cookie" and cheerfully head off to the gym or select a different food on the menu.

But remember, the most important shield of all is not someone else. Your most important shield of all is your Success File! That's where you will need to go when your codreamers are busy or stuck in negative spaces themselves. Or when you have already exceeded what your codreamers believe is possible. Your Success File is where you need to go when all else fails. In there is all the support you will need to pick up your shield, rebuild your self-confidence and keep heading toward your outcome. That's where you will find recorded all the thousands of steps you have already taken. Those completed steps are there to remind you that you can self-confidently keep going.

You are the only one who can shift you to 3rd gear

Don't wait for your expert to shift you into 3rd gear. The shift to 3rd gear is one you must make yourself, in your own timing... in an unexpected moment when you have an Aha! Or when you wake up realizing, Wow, I just thought of a new approach. A creative new way that will not only help me but also others. Or when, Aha! you experience someone else's dream you choose to co-hologram and co-own.

You need to become powerful codreamers of others' dreams too. You are the only one who can *decide* whether you are willing to set aside old fears and beliefs, so you can learn new information that can move you ahead in new directions... the directions you want to go.

You need to know more to lose more!

Knowledge is a powerful shield! To enhance the power of your shield, you need to increase your knowledge base. The more you know, the easier it will be to fight off unfounded negativity and disagreement. Greater knowledge gives you greater certainty and persistence. More staying power and accuracy!

Some of the ideas we introduce may seem too new or too outlandish, or too old or too old-fashioned. But what if they work?

What if using them could change your weight and health... especially if you've already tried every diet you've ever heard of? So stay open to what comes next. Suspend judgment and let the information sink in," smiled Susan.

Heads up... You're wired *not* to lose weight. Is wheat worse than sodas? Beware of The Addictive Mix!

One of the 10 success skills HSPs use consistently is "commit to your outcome and stay flexible about method." Instead of getting stuck in how it's been done before, HSPs are open to new ideas and approaches. They don't care about being right, they care about getting results. And hopefully so do you.

Historically humans lived shorter lives

We walked. We worked. We went to bed when it got dark. We ate off the land. And we died early.

Hunger and stress... primitive man risked getting eaten

In primitive times, humans were hunters. We went out to kill a rabbit, pheasant, elephant, tiger or lion. Hunting was treacherous, we could be eaten by the very animal we were hunting. All this stress made us hungry. And that was important.

Getting hungry was essential to early man. There was no refrigeration and plenty of animals nearby who wanted to eat the same food we did. Stress hormones allowed early man to have ravenous enough appetites to eat their whole kill before it spoiled or was dragged away. Then, of course, early man also realized they would probably not eat meat again for weeks.

Berries, nuts and roots, yes, but during that undefined number of weeks, early man might have to resort to eating leaves and bark. The appendix, which we usually remove, was the organ that allowed them to digest these not-so-desirable meat substitutes.

Most Egyptians lived to be about 30. In the Middle Ages if you were 40 you were considered to be ancient!

50% of people died before 20 in the Middle Ages

In the Middle Ages, 33% of babies died before they were two. 50% of young people died before they were 20. Many women died in childbirth. Many men died in wars. But those who survived often lived to be 60, 70 or older. There are parish registries of people who lived to be over 100. People in the Middle Ages had it in them to live long lives, but, like many of us, circumstances got in the way.

Where does the U.S. rank in longevity?

If you live in Swaziland today, your life expectancy is 31 years. If you live in Angola, it is 38. If you live in Monaco, it is 89.73. In Israel, it is 80.96. In the U.S., it is 78.37 and with the obesity rate increasing, this number may go down even more. Amazing, isn't it? Here we are living in the richest country on earth, yet we don't have the greatest health and longevity.[23]

Today we can easily live 20 or 30 years beyond retirement. But the real question is... do we want to live those years obese with heart disease and diabetes, or do we want to be healthy and enjoying full lives? These extra years are presenting an opportunity and a challenge few people have had historically. Will we be healthy, wealthy and wise? Or will we be unhealthy, financially-strapped and obese?

Stress makes us hungry-enough-to-eat-it-all up. And that can be deadly

We live in a world where perceived stress levels are high. Work demands and family demands. Phone calls, emails and texts. Meetings and workouts. And we take work-stress with us wherever we go... thanks or no thanks to cell phones and laptops.

Today we can stop at a restaurant, drive-through, fast food, takeout, or convenience store on almost any corner and, for 5 or 6 dollars, purchase more calories, sodium and fat than our ancestors probably ate in months. Cheaper and more convenient but far more life-threatening in other ways. Obesity, heart disease, diabetes, arthritis and more... forget about lions and tigers, these diseases are far more dangerous and lethal long term.

Man spent thousands of years starving

They starved and then they feasted. And then they starved again.

It turns out the body God designed for us is still trying to prevent starvation by holding on to fat stores we no longer need.

Today's stress is making us ravenous enough to eat whatever we can buy. But there's no kill and no long distance trek. And few calories are burned in the process of finding food today.

Our factory system of eating and exercising

We don't eat and exercise the way early man did, planting, hunting and harvesting as seasons and circumstances required.

Today we have rigorous work-schedules, drop-off times for our kids, lunch appointments and agreed-upon dinner times. And we have rigorous workout schedules, regular days and times when we do classes and workouts, when we attempt to burn as many calories as we eat or more. Or we try to do all of our exercise on the weekend. The weekend warrior.

With regular routines, chances are you are gaining weight

Yes, that was really surprising to me when I first heard it. But it's true. You can't fool your body but it may be fooling you into keeping on weight. Why? *Because you're too consistent*.

Even food-conscious triathletes are heavy these days. In this chapter we will look at why. And the reasons are surprising.

You and your body have different outcomes in mind

You want to lose fat but your body wants to hold on to it... just in case. Just in case all the grocery stores in your neighborhood close and all the restaurants as well. And all the convenience stores. But no, these days there is next to no chance that you'll die of starvation as long as you stay healthy.

Body priority... burn carbs first, glycogen second, and third fat

In her New York Times bestselling book, *Crack the Fat-Loss Code* and her latest *Conquer the Fat-Loss Code*, nutrition expert Wendy Chant presents vital information about how our body's starvation-prevention mechanism works. This is information you need to know now. Information that will successfully guide you through weight-loss plateaus.

Your body has a priority system. First, it uses carbs. Second, it burns glycogen stored in your muscles and liver. Third, only when glycogen stores are low, it burns excess fat in your body.

Carbohydrate is the most important source of energy for exercise. Carbs provide the energy to fuel muscles and are broken down into smaller sugars (glucose, fructose and galactose) that get absorbed and used as energy. Any glucose not immediately needed gets stored in your muscles and liver in the form of glycogen. *Once glycogen stores are full, any extra gets converted to fat.*

Because glycogen is immediately accessible, it is used for short, intense bouts of exercise from sprinting to weight lifting. During long, slow exercise, fat can provide fuel, but glycogen is still needed to breakdown fat into something your muscles can use.

If the body doesn't have enough carbohydrate, glycogen or fat, protein will be broken down to make glucose for energy. But protein's primary role is to build and rebuild muscles, bone, skin, hair and other tissues so relying on it for energy could limit your ability to maintain your tissues and health.

72 /48 rule for getting rid of excess fat

God gave us a starvation-prevention mechanism most of us haven't understood so it's been working against us. Here are the basics.

72 IN...

Every 72 hours (3 days) your body assesses how much food you are taking in and calculates how it can reserve as much energy as possible... just in case.

48 OUT...

Every 48 hours (2 days) your body adjusts the amount of energy it is using... *assuming you will keep expending as much energy as you have in the previous 48 hours...* so it can keep functioning. *Your body then decides whether to convert energy to fat or burn fat to create energy.*[24]

This formula worked for early man but it may *not* be working for us, given our scheduled lives and routines. We're highly predictable so our bodies have figured out how to keep us at the weight we are now. And when we go on diets, our body quickly figures them out too and our weight loss plateaus.

When you go on your diet, your body thinks you're starving

"Remember, the minute your body thinks you're on a diet, it will do *anything and everything it can* to hold on to as much fat as possible because it senses you are going into *starvation mode*. Your brain will send the rest of your body a signal to conserve energy for the coming dry spell. It shuts down body temperature, reduces the absorption rate of food, and slows down your metabolism, all with the intention of storing more fat so it will have plenty of energy *just in case*," says Chant.

You are like a bear fattening up before it hibernates so it will have enough energy to make it till spring. But there's no hibernation.

How to move past Weight Loss Plateaus

"Once your body learns to survive by calculating how to store what you give it and expend less, your diet plateaus. This 'sticking point' is failure for the dieter but victory for the body," says Chant. She has shown that dieters can easily break a weight loss plateau, lose unwanted fat and keep it off for life by Macro-Patterning.

Trick your body into burning fat!

Macro-patterning lowers your glycogen levels (reduces your carb intake) a few days a week just enough to tell your body to burn stored fat. The next day it rebuilds the glycogen level (by eating carbs) so your body doesn't go into fat-conserving mode. And you don't feel you're being deprived of starches and fruits or you'll never be able to eat your favorite foods that could send you off into eating jags.

Cycling carb days and protein days. And pigging out every 18 days!

Chant says cycling carb and protein days tricks your body into losing fat because it doesn't have a chance to adapt to the way you are eating. She suggests restricting carbs on certain days and eating them on others. And, pigging out every 18 days, especially if your metabolism is super sluggish. On that day, go crazy and eat whatever you want.

Susan has found Macro-Patterning to be easy and effective. "I eat the same foods in the same quantities as I did before, just on different days. I'm "macro-patterning" my exercise too, alternating weight-training and cardio instead of doing the same workout every day. And the fat around my middle is finally melting away. I wasn't heavy but my body had its energy reserves stored there and I couldn't exercise them off no matter how hard I tried." .

Thermogenic foods… burn more calories without more exercise

Most foods are thermogenic, that is, they produce heat when you digest them. But some foods are more thermogenic than others.

Let's get our vocabulary straight before we begin. *Thermogenic* means tending to produce *heat* from the Greek word *thermos*. And *calor,* which is the root of the word *calorie,* comes from the Latin, Spanish and Portuguese word *calor* and also means heat. So whichever word we use, we are talking about heat.

Every time you eat, some of the calories you consume are used for chewing, swallowing, absorbing, metabolizing and eliminating. Bottom line, for processing that food.

Some foods produce more heat than others

These more-heat-producing foods are referred to as Thermogenic foods because they require more calories to consume, digest, metabolize and eliminate than others do. And they heat up your metabolism more in the process.

On average, the thermic effect of food is about 10 percent of your caloric intake. If you consume 2,000 calories, you expend about 200 calories processing it. By eating more Thermogenic foods you burn more calories and, bottom line, you can lose a pound or two a month without doing anything other than digesting your food.

Fats are easily processed so they only have a thermic effect of 3 percent. That is, you only burn 3 calories to digest 100 calories of fat. Fruit and fibrous vegetables have a higher thermic effect, about 20 percent. So you burn about *20 calories to process 100 calories of fruit and vegetables*.

When I was growing up in Brazil they ate lots of thermogenic foods like... cinnamon, acai berries, fish, lean chicken and hot spices. Spices like cinnamon, nutmeg, cloves and cayenne.

Zero-calorie spices like cinnamon, nutmeg, cloves and cayenne can increase your metabolism *by as much as 78 percent*. And all you need is a pill that contains it or about a half teaspoon on your oatmeal or in your applesauce.

By all means, include thermogenic foods in your diet. Every little bit of added heat helps.

Protein increases your metabolic rate by 36 percent

Your metabolism is the process by which your body converts calories into energy. When you eat protein, your body burns five times as many calories as when you eat carbohydrates and fat. *Protein increases your metabolic rate by 36 per cent*, or to say it differently, it takes 36 calories to digest 100 calories of protein.

Choose protein you chew, like lean red meat, chicken, turkey and eggs. How do you know how many grams of protein you're eating? When you buy a product, the Nutrition Fact Label will tell you how many grams of protein are contained in a serving. How much and what kinds of protein we should be eating is a matter of heated discussion we will talk about in much more detail later.

Deceivingly "Diet"... thought you'd be interested in this

Here is a Pop Quiz from *Prevention Magazine*. "What's the single biggest source of calories for Americans? White bread? Big Macs? Actually, try soda. The average American drinks about two cans of the stuff every day. "But I drink diet soda," you say. "With no calories or sugar, it's the perfect alternative for weight watchers...Right?" Not so fast. Before you pop the top off the caramel-colored bubbly, know this: guzzling diet soda comes with its own set of side effects.[25]

Seven side effects of diet soda

1. Diet soda is bad for your kidneys. 2. Diet soda is linked to 34% higher risk of metabolic syndrome which includes belly fat and high cholesterol. 3. A University of Texas Health Science Center study found that downing two or more cans a day increased waistlines by 500%. 4. Cocktails made with diet soda get you drunker, faster. 5. Diet sodas contain mold inhibitors that can

cause severe damage to DNA in the mitochondria and totally inactivate it. Diet sodas have also been linked to hives, asthma and other allergic conditions. 6. Diet sodas are very acidic and can dissolve tooth enamel. 7. Soft drink cans are coated with BPA which has been linked to everything from heart disease to obesity to reproductive problems.

"Unfortunately, diet soda is more in vogue than ever. Kids consume the stuff at more than double the rate of last decade, according to research in the American Journal of Clinical Nutrition. Among adults, consumption has grown almost 25%. But knowing these 7 side effects of drinking diet soda may help you kick the can for good."[26]

An interesting possibility… give up artificial sweeteners and lose 5 pounds in a month!

Artificial sweeteners *do not* raise core body temperature to boost metabolism the way other foods do. They do the opposite; they are *non-thermogenic*. According to research from Purdue University, "When you eat them, you actually lower your metabolism… which sabotages your weight loss goals," says Chant. To test this theory, she asked eight avid diet soda drinkers to give up them up for a month. Without any other change, they each lost five pounds that month.[27]

Urban Myth: Negative Calorie Foods

Some sources say some foods burn more calories than they contain. They call these foods Negative Calorie foods and they usually include celery, berries, broccoli, cabbage, apples, pears and leafy greens like spinach and lettuce.

This is a myth, but it does reveal an exciting reality. Most thermogenic foods are high-fiber, low-calorie fruits and vegetables and you use 20% of their calories just to digest them. In addition, their fiber slows digestion down, stabilizes blood sugar and reduces your appetite. Apples and pears do even more.

An apple a day isn't simply something your grandmother used to say

Apples, berries and other fresh fruits contain pectin in their skins. Pectin is a carbohydrate that has no calories and is a source of fiber, a prime ingredient in a healthy diet. Pectin limits the amount of fat your cells can absorb. Also pectin causes your stomach to empty more slowly so you feel satisfied longer. This means you will ultimately eat less, leading to weight loss.

Truly negative calories… green tea, hot peppers and spices

Green tea is a truly negative calorie food. Green tea has no calories and it produces a powerful thermogenic effect. Green tea contains catechins which appear to increase your metabolic rate. In a 12-week study, subjects who drank green tea lost 7 pounds more than those who ate the same diet but didn't drink green tea.

After eating red hot chili or spicy hot wings, have you ever noticed beads of sweat breaking out on your forehead? Capsaicin, found in cayenne, habaneros and most chili peppers, raises your body temperature. No, capsaicin isn't going to make you sweat the way hot yoga or a sauna would, but it will raise your metabolism 8% for a couple of hours. And that's not bad.

Cortisol and Adrenal Fatigue… stress makes you gain weight

When you're stressed, your adrenal glands release a hormone called cortisol, which slows down your metabolism and increases your appetite, making you more vulnerable than usual to grabbing high-calorie comfort foods which will increase belly fat and your risk of heart disease and diabetes… even greater stresses. So to re-establish a healthy weight you need to minimize your stress and learn how to use exercise and breathing to handle the rest.

Lack of sleep can make you gain

We need about 7 1/2 hours of sleep a night, but today many people are getting far less. The way reduced sleep impacts your weight involves two important hormones… ghrelin and leptin.

Here's a weight-loss formula you will want to remember.

more ghrelin + less leptin = weight gain

Here's why.

> *Ghrelin is the hormone that tells your body start eating*
> *Leptin is the hormone that tells your body stop eating*

Ghrelin plays a positive role in our health. It creates the sensations that urge us to stop what we're doing and refuel so we don't get exhausted, make mistakes, get injured or lose too much weight and muscle. When food reaches the stomach, ghrelin levels drop quickly and stay low until about an hour before the next meal is typically eaten.

When you are sleep deprived, you have more ghrelin (start eating) than leptin (stop eating.) in your system. So when you're sleep-deprived you tend to overeat. Your metabolism is slower and the heat in your body is less.

The Addictive Mix... fat, salt and sugar

America is fat and getting fatter. In our effort to improve on God's miraculous foods, we have inadvertently taken apart foods that worked for thousands of years and reconstructed them into foods that are cheap and easy to produce but *that are now making us obese and killing us*.

Remember the dumpster diving former head of the FDA, Dr. David Kessler, who finally emerged with his prize... ingredient labels spelling out the *fats, salt and sugar* in Chili's Southwestern Eggrolls, Boneless Shanghai Wings? Here's more.

In a new study published in the *Journal of Clinical Endocrinology and Metabolism*, researchers found that high-fat foods, like fast foods, raised ghrelin levels and increased hunger. Eating carbohydrates made people even hungrier.

Only *proteins* lowered ghrelin levels substantially and helped tame hunger pangs. No doubt that's why early man was so eager to find meat. That's why I eat a protein snack after I work out. Three hours after your workout is your muscle-making window. I recommend eating protein before you workout too.

Michael Bloomberg on obesity

On CNN, New York City Mayor Michael Bloomberg said, "the single biggest public health issue of our day is obesity." Then he continued making powerful-point after powerful-point: the average family of four is rapidly approaching 1,000 pounds. Yes, a family of four! Six-year-olds are being diagnosed with Type 2

Diabetes never before seen at that age. The blood of 19 year olds looks like that of 60 year olds.

"Over the last few years obesity has become a bigger and bigger problem, not just in the United States but around the world. I think this is the first year in the history of the world when more people will die from the effects of too much food than from starvation. Also we think it's the first disease in the history of the world that has gone from being a rich person's disease to a poor person's disease."

In New York City, thanks to Bloomberg, they now have smoking bans and big-sugary-drink bans. Here's the big difference. "If you smoke and I'm in the same room, I get hurt. If you and I are in the same room and you are obese, I don't get hurt short term, but I do have to eventually pay your medical bills, because that's actually what happens."[28] Obesity is a personal health issue and a public health issue as well.

On September 13, 2012, The New York City Board of Health voted to approve Mayor Michael R. Bloomberg's ban on the sale of large sodas and other sugary drinks at restaurants, street carts and movie theaters. This is the first restriction of its kind in the country. Bravo, New York City![29]

Is wheat an even bigger threat than sodas and sugar?

But could there be something even more devastating to the public? According to Dr. William Davis, author of *Wheat Belly, a New York Times* bestseller, "There is no question that, at least for some people, especially younger people, sugar exposure in soft drinks, junk foods, and snacks is a big problem." But Davis has an important suggestion, "*Switch the order...* when you eliminate all wheat the desire for sweets is nearly always markedly reduced, since the *appetite-stimulating gliadin protein of wheat* is now gone. It is a far easier task to eliminate wheat first, rather than to eliminate sugars first."[30]

Two slices of whole wheat bread raise blood sugar more than two tablespoons of table sugar, more than some candy bars! This has been known since the Glycemic Index was invented in 1981, even though the nutrition community is still encouraging us to eat more whole grains.

"Eat more wheat, and blood sugar increases in magnitude and frequency. This leads to higher and more frequent rises in insulin, which, in turn, creates insulin resistance, the condition that leads to diabetes," says Davis.

Repeated high blood sugars damage pancreatic beta cells that produce insulin. These beta cells have very little ability to regenerate so when they are damaged repeatedly, fewer and fewer healthy beta cells are left to produce insulin and blood sugar levels remain high.

"So the wheat we are advised to eat more of is not the solution to the diabetes epidemic that is expected to include *one in two Americans in the near future, and 346 million people worldwide* — eating more 'healthy whole grains' is, I believe, the *cause* of this situation. And removing it sets us back on a course to stop or even reverse it," urges Davis.

Think about it... bread, pancakes, muffins, croutons, pasta, pizza, cookies, pastries, pies, thickeners and extenders. Visible and invisible, wheat has managed to find its way into almost every product we eat, every restaurant and kitchen. Check a few labels in your cupboard and you'll see. But, depending on your age, "today's wheat" may not be the wheat you grew up loving.[31]

Wheat: From Promised Land to Promised Productivity

For thousands of years wheat had been a food staple and its DNA remained virtually the same… until 1985. Wheat has been central to religious rituals of major religions. Moses' Promised Land was "a land of wheat, barley and vineyards," The wafer representing the body of Jesus is wheat. Wheat is holy for Muslims as well; it is stored standing up and never thrown away in public. Wheat ground with sand chipped the Egyptians' teeth but nevertheless fed them well. Wheat was such an important food staple that it was brought to the New World by Columbus, to New England by Gosnold, to Mexico and the U.S. southwest by Spanish explorers.

Wheat had virtually the same DNA for thousands of years… from its discovery and early cultivation about 8,500 BC by a semi-nomadic tribe called Natufians who improvised a way to prevent starvation between animal kills by growing a very early variety of the grain we now call wheat. Early wheat was coarsely ground and cooked into porridge or a flattened cake. In Egypt thousands of years later, finely ground wheat, yeast and leavenings came into use, and voila… the first loaf of bread.

As man evolved, there is convincing evidence that switching to a grain-based diet caused humans to become shorter, fatter and sicker, even in pre-biblical times. If the hunt failed and you are starving, eat wheat by all means. But Dr. Jared Diamond points out this *early convenience food* had adverse health consequences even then (bone disease, dental decay, cancer, perhaps atherosclerosis.) As long ago as 100 AD, there were descriptions of the ravages of Celiac Disease, an extreme wheat intolerance.

"It's the changes introduced by geneticists over the past 40-50 years, *coupled with dietary advice to consume more wheat*, that have conspired to create this current mess we are in, turning wheat from a problem ingredient into a health scourge exerting adverse health effects on an international scale," says. Davis.

What happened to wheat 40 to 50 years ago? DNA changes

With worldwide population and hunger increasing, with new production techniques and bio-engineering, scientists decided to make changes in the DNA of wheat. From fields full of four foot tall "amber waves of grain" to today's mechanized fields of 18" stocky stalks of bio-wheat. A farmer's dream... easier to cut and harvest. A food supplier's dream... cheaper and more productive. Despite all these changes in DNA and appearance, it kept the same name... wheat. New and improved, but still wheat. Or is it?

Susan loved to bake crusty golden-topped braided breads

"This *new wheat* story really hit home. My home. I have a long delicious history of baking bread for my family and friends, adding granular yeast to "baby bath" water and letting it bubble, adding milk, sugar, butter and a touch of salt, kneading in enough flour till it formed a smooth elastic ball, till it doubled in a warm bowl, till I punched it down, braided it and let it rise again. Then the aroma from my oven called in my hungry kids and neighbor's kids as well.

But all that ended when I developed a devastating allergy to wheat. Guess when? About 1985. And I haven't been able to eat those golden, crusty egg-yolk-coated, sesame-seed-topped loaves. Or even touch that elastic dough without severe allergic reactions. And my daughter is allergic too," added Susan.

Marc's story... a home united, a kitchen divided

"My 10 year-old grandson Marc is one of the smartest kids I know (except for his older brother Sam, of course.) Marc can tell you everything about every sports team, player and stat, whether it's soccer, baseball or football. He amazes his teachers with his broad knowledge-base and astounding memory. He does macro photography with me and achieves pin-point focus. And Marc does something else that always melts my heart.

Marc is so full of life and energy that it's hard for him to stay still, even when we watch TV. He sits. He stands. He rolls around on the floor. But as fidgety as Marc is, every time I visit him there's a very special moment when he invisibly slides into my lap and snuggles up with me. I never even notice he's there until he's wound his way around my heart. Needless to say I adore these special moments with Marc.

But Marc's house is divided. No, they're all very close and have lots of fun together so that's not what I mean. Marc's house is divided because he, his brother and father eat pizza, cakes, cookies and bread, but his mother, my daughter Margaret, can't. His home's kitchen drawers are divided, too. Gluten-free flours like tapioca, rice and potato starch are in one area and regular flour in another. And never the two shall meet or Margaret will get sick or I will if I'm there for one of Marc's Dad's famous gourmet meals. Like Mom and Dad, Sam and Marc are both good cooks and well-informed about gluten and gluten-free. And they know how to bake muffins, cakes, pizzas and cobblers both ways. Because they need to," added Susan.

From yesterday's fields of four foot tall "amber waves of grain" to today's mechanized fields of high-yielding, easy-to-harvest, 18" stocky stalks of bio-grain which are producing painful and sometimes life-threatening allergies. And that Dr. William Davis suspects may be a key reason for America's obesity which has dramatically soared since, guess when? 1985.

The law of unintended consequences applies

"A loaf of bread, biscuit, or pancake of today is different than its counterpart of a thousand years ago, different even from what our grandmothers made. It might look the same, even taste much the same, but there are biochemical differences. *Small changes in wheat protein's structure* can spell the difference between a devastating immune response to wheat protein versus no immune response at all," writes Dr. Davis.

It was assumed their "new wheat" would be an equally good food staple, but *the developers missed an essential step*. "No animal or human safety testing was conducted on the new genetic strains that were created." Since then, it has been found that their "new wheat" contains "a higher quantity of genes for gluten proteins that are associated with Celiac Disease.

New York Times: Celiac four times more frequent than 1950s

Tara Parker-Pope wrote in the *New York Times* July 2, 2009, "While it's been known that the incidence of Celiac is on the rise, it hasn't been clear whether doctors are simply looking for it more often, and therefore finding more cases. But new research from the Mayo Clinic in Rochester, Minnesota, suggests that the disease is four times more common today than in the 1950s, and not just because doctors are more likely to test for it.

The study in the journal *Gastroenterology*, analyzed blood samples collected from 9,133 healthy adults collected at Warren Air Force Base between 1948 and 1954. Another 12,768 gender-matched subjects from a study in Olmsted County, Minnesota, were also analyzed for signs of Celiac Disease. Of the blood samples collected 50 years ago, only 0.2 percent had Celiac Disease. In the more recent blood samples, the incidence of

Celiac Disease was more than four times greater. Today, it's estimated that about one in 100 people have Celiac Disease."[32]

What is Celiac Disease? How do you know whether you have it?

If you have Celiac Disease, when you eat gluten your body attacks itself trying to get rid of the gluten and damages your small intestine in the process. This does not occur in non-celiac individuals.

When you look at the wall of the small intestine through a microscope, what you see looks like a shag rug. The shaggy projections, or villi, greatly expand the absorptive area of the small intestine. The solution to Celiac Disease is to avoid eating wheat altogether. If you don't avoid it, there can be a slow, gradual blunting of the villi. And a slow gradual blunting of your ability to absorb the nutrients you eat and need.

Thousands of children die from undiagnosed Celiac Disease. An article entitled, *The Global Burden of Childhood Coeliac Disease: A Neglected Component of Diarrhoeal Mortality* states: "In 2010 there were around 2.2 million children under 5 years of age living with Celiac Disease. Among these children there could be 42,000 deaths related to Celiac Disease annually."[33]

Symptoms of wheat intolerance or wheat sensitivity

Celiac Disease is the most extreme form of gluten intolerance. But there are thousands, or is it millions, of other people who suffer from wheat intolerance. To eliminate your symptoms, you may want to eliminate wheat too. Common symptoms caused by wheat sensitivity include: bloating, constipation, diarrhea, skin problems, pale foul-smelling stool, fatty stool, depression, anxiety, joint pain, chronic fatigue, bloating, weight loss, iron deficiency (anemia), malnutrition, tingling in the hands and feet, fertility problems and missed periods, canker sores in the mouth.

How can you learn whether you have Celiac Disease?

If you are concerned, your doctor can test you for Celiac Disease using a skin test or blood test. What if your tests come back negative? It's possible to have a wheat sensitivity that doesn't show up on skin or blood tests. If so, you can use a food elimination diet (that means you can eliminate wheat, all wheat) to find out whether, or not, it is creating your symptoms.

Fortunately today there are many "I can't believe it's not wheat" substitutes which are not only delicious but easily available. Many restaurants offer gluten-free menus as well.

We are trying to cope with the health consequences this "new wheat" is causing, but shouldn't we also be looking to change the wheat we plant and harvest? To un-modify the DNA or plant heritage seeds? Or to eliminate wheat from our diets and find healthier choices?

Even churches are aware of gluten intolerance

The Roman Catholic Church says the wafer for the Eucharist must be "wheaten bread." It permits low-gluten bread for celiacs even though the dietary recommendation is to avoid gluten altogether. Many Protestant churches offer communicants gluten-free bread or a rice-based cracker.

Your Knowledge Base is a powerful shield

Just because something worked for thousands of years doesn't' mean it works the same way today. Just because a food has the same name... wheat, tomato, chicken or beef... doesn't mean it contains the same nutrients. We need to keep asking questions and expanding our Knowledge Base... the information we have available to us. We need to keep updating the experts we use... and the information they can provide to us. We need to keep shielding ourselves with up to date successes and information.

In a world that is changing as rapidly as this one, we need to do our very best to stay on top of what is going on so we can maintain our health and balance, our children's and our planet's.

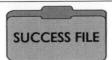

SUCCESS FILE

Time to Success File again...
Diet Skill Eight: Shielding... building your Knowledge Base

What did you learn in this skill that will be useful to you or someone you codream with? What new information did you gain and how will you use it?

Might wheat be a factor in your weight gain? Do you have the symptoms of wheat sensitivity? Does anyone else you know?

How about The Addictive Mix? What are you addicted to eating that you need to change to lose weight? What is your plan for doing that now?

Do you eat the same foods and exercise the same way day after day? How can you disrupt that pattern so you can lose weight?

How can you trick your body into burning fat?

Have you been getting enough sleep? How can you get more?

Are you constantly tired and burned out? Have you had your hormone levels checked recently? What is your cortisol level?

What thermogenic foods and spices are you eating... like cinnamon, salsa or hot peppers for example? Have you tried adding green tea to your diet?

Turn to the back of the book and add as many more Successes as you can. When you Success File is full... you know the rest!

Diet Skill Nine: Committing to Outcome... instead of hanging on to familiar methods

Have we gotten our outcomes and our methods confused? In the 1st gear of life when we were beginning to learn, we were told what to do, but not why to do it. When we got to be three-years old that famous childhood question popped up, why? Why, Mommy? Why, Daddy? Why, why, why... what is my outcome? Tell me. Tell me.

Why is outcome. And *how* is method. From time to time, as adults, we seem to return to our old outcome versus method confusion. We hear ourselves saying "we have to do it this way" or "this is the way we have always done it" instead of asking ourselves "what do we want instead?" Instead of gearing up into creativity to find new approaches.

Have we given up nutritional value for the sake of convenience?

Have we abandoned our personal and global outcome... which is to provide healthy, nourishing food for our population... so our manufacturers can make huge profits? At whose cost? At the cost of each of us and our families? At the cost of our economy and nation?

We've de-constructed foods. Can we re-construct and re-store them?

Isn't it time now for us to use our brains to begin healing and remedying what we have un-done? To begin to work to understand and respect the reasons why God's foods were created the way they were, to heal the destruction we have done to our bodies and health. Our soil and bees. Our planet and atmosphere. To begin to supplement and support our bodies in healing.

Commit to your holographic outcome and your Razz will go to work for you, waking you in the night or zinging you in the aisle or when someone is in the elevator you need to meet.

Commit to the outcome you have pre-experienced and play it over and over, reinforcing its details and amplifying its power, adding or subtracting details to update Your hologram as new information comes in. Remember, the more detail, the attractive power your hologram has. Then trust your God-Given Miraculous Brain to guide you there. This is the formula I observed inventors and innovators using, and trusting consistently.

Like those surgery patients, it's vital to your health to have a detailed, attractive future hologram in mind. A destination you're looking forward to enjoying. Something to keep you going on your weight loss/health gain program, something powerful like going to my daughter's wedding is for me. Of course at that moment, I will probably already be planning for my grandchildren, their Baby Namings and Bar Mitzvahs. I will already be updating my future hologram to make it more attractive and enticing.

OK Susan, I now see that committing to outcome instead of hanging on to familiar methods is another one of the 10 success skills I was using without realizing it.

To commit to outcome and stay flexible about method, you will need to gear up whenever your Razz alerts you, or your codreamers' Razzes alert them on your behalf. Keep *why* in sight and don't get stuck in *how*. Pay attention to realities and don't get stuck in *old ways*. Or startling new ones. Believe it or not, like it or not, comfortable or not, your Razz may be taking you into breakthrough and creativity. Into uncertainty and new territory. Into 3rd gear!

So fasten your seat belt as we slosh back and forth... meat/no meat, dairy/no dairy, wheat/no wheat, high carbs/low carbs, and as we consider the impact of blood types on an individual's diet. Do you know your blood type? It may make a big difference in finding what works best for you. Keep your mind open to consider new ideas and ancient ones.

The opinions expressed here are strong ones (pioneers tend to be very passionate about their discoveries) so you will probably feel yourself being blown one way and then another. But stay in your seat till we hear all their voices and their challengers' voices as well, as we work to find a food balance that suits you uniquely.

Which protein is better? Animal or plant?

"Let me start by saying that when I saw the movie *Forks Over Knives*, I was stunned and impressed by what Campbell and Esselstyn presented about the dangers of animal protein and the virtues of a plant-based diet.

As someone who looks like an unwatered flower when I don't get enough protein, I was shaken to my roots and eager to learn more about their research and sort through their strong conclusions. Here is the *Forks Over Knives* story followed by questions other researchers have raised about their work," added Susan.

Two doctors who believed in milk and beef were forced to change their minds

Dr. Colin Campbell and Dr. Caldwell Esselstyn are prominent doctors who spent their boyhoods on dairy farms in different states. Each believed, with all his fiber, that milk was the *perfect* food and meat the *perfect* protein. But their global life experiences in nutrition and medicine forced them to change their minds and diets. Their experiences pressed them into the joys and discomforts of 3rd gear Break-through and discovery.

Instead of feeding cattle, Campbell took on feeding starving children

As a nutritional biochemist at Cornell University, Campbell was focused on feeding and growing healthy livestock. But with millions of starving, malnourished children in our world, his focus began to shift. How can we feed these children and *make sure they get enough protein*?

In Campbell's mind and the nutritional community's mind at the time, *protein* meant *animal protein*. The idea that plants provide protein was a little-considered possibility. But when he was developing food programs in the Philippines in the 60s, Campbell realized feeding animal protein to millions of children was far too expensive. So to keep down costs, he decided to feed them plant protein instead. "When you are eating whole foods, it's virtually impossible to be protein deficient without being calorie deficient," declared Campbell. "Because even if you take foods that have the least protein in them, let's say potatoes or rice for example, 8 or 9 % protein is the figure we need more or less."

Next Campbell stumbled on something that changed his protein-thinking drastically. Children of affluent Filipino families who could afford to eat high levels of animal protein were mysteriously developing liver cancer. Since liver cancer is rare in kids, Campbell knew these observations were significant, but not why.[34]

Remember how your Razz alerted you to buy toothpaste when you were at the grocery store. Aha, there it is. Well, your Razz will alert you about anything you have in mind... especially an unfolding mystery.

Dr. Campbell's Razz and an obscure Indian study

Soon after, Campbell was reading an article in an obscure Indian journal about a rat study and cancer when his Razz alerted him, Aha, there it is! First researchers exposed rats to daily doses of aflatoxin, a carcinogen. Then they fed them a diet of casein (an isolated milk protein) in two different concentrations: *20% of total calories* turned cancer on and *5% of total calories* turned cancer off.

First, those liver cancers in children of affluent Filipino families, now the Indian study. Reality was shifting in Campbell's mind.

20 percent animal protein turned cancer on, but 20% plant protein did not

Returning to Cornell, Campbell worked to replicate the Indian study. When he fed rats 20% animal protein tumor* growth exploded at the end of 3 weeks. When he switched their diets to 5% animal protein*, tumor growth went down. (Note: We have added these asterisks and they will be discussed later)

Campbell noticed something else... 20 percent animal protein* turned cancer on, *but 20% plant protein from soy beans and wheat did not*. Despite what Campbell thought growing up on a dairy farm, despite his longstanding belief that milk was "the perfect food," despite the authoritative advice of the National Dairy Council and The American Dietetic Association, animal protein didn't look *perfect* to Campbell any more. His life was forever changed. And so was his diet.

Campbell wanted a large scale population study and found it in China

In 1974, Chinese Premier Zhou Enlai, knowing he had terminal bladder cancer, decided to give his country a broader understanding of cancer. He initiated one of the largest and most comprehensive cancer studies in history. Between 1973 and 1975, 650,000 researchers catalogued mortality patterns in every county in China, over 880 million people. After his death, the results were published in a book entitled *Cancer Atlas*.

When Dr. Junshi Chen, senior research director for China's Center for Disease Control, visited Cornell he met Campbell and a major collaboration began. They travelled together to China to do further research. Finally in 1990, 10 years later, Campbell, Chen and associates published *Diet, Lifestyle and Cancer in China*.

Plant-food-based diet associated with lower death rates

Chen proclaimed… "The major message we got… is only one message: *A plant food based diet*, of mainly cereal grains, vegetables and fruits *and very little animal food* is always associated with lower mortality of certain cancers, stroke and coronary heart disease."

Jane E. Brody of *The New York Times* wrote, "Early findings from the most comprehensive large study ever taken of the relationships between diet and the risk of developing disease are challenging much of American dietary dogma. The study, being conducted in China, paints a bold portrait of a plant-based eating plan that is more likely to promote health than disease."[35]

In Hawaii, Dr. McDougall was noticing another pattern

In the 1970s, while Dr. John McDougall was practicing medicine on a Hawaiian sugar plantation, he started noticing that the longer immigrants from Japan, the Philippines, Korea and China lived in Hawaii, the sicker they got. The first generation was trim, healthy and vital even into their 80s and 90s. But their kids got fat and sick. And their grandchildren got fatter and sicker still.

The diet was the difference

"The first generation had learned a diet of rice and vegetables in their native land, but their kids started to give up the rice and replace it with animal foods, dairy products, meats, and the results were obvious. They got fat and sick so I knew at that point what caused most diseases," says McDougall.

Though McDougall doesn't say so here, the longer these immigrants were in Hawaii the more they were moving toward a Western Diet which includes not only much more meat but also more wheat and processed foods than traditionally eaten in their homelands.

Was it animal protein or was it our Western Diet… more meat, more dairy, more sugar, more wheat?

In the early 20th century, Americans on average were eating 120 pounds of meat and 29 pounds of dairy a year. By 2007 we were eating 222 pounds of meat and 605 pounds of dairy a year! With the surge of convenience and fast foods, sugar consumption soared dramatically during those years too, from 40 pounds a year in 1913 to 156 pounds total refined sweeteners in 2012.[36] (And 138.1 pounds of wheat in 2007.)

In the late 50's, the American diet began to make a sharp turn from home-cooked, farm-raised foods to burgers and drive-ins, supermarkets and convenience foods... packaged soups, sauces, breads and TV dinners. Up, up, and away, more-better-faster. America was in 2nd gear!

Nixon declared War on Cancer but not America's accelerating food changes

Twice as much meat, 20 times more dairy, 4 times more sugar... and cancer was on the rise in the U.S. too. In 1971 President Nixon declared War on Cancer, *but not on these accelerating food changes.*

While food manufacturers are profiting, we are paying a high price. "Obesity, diabetes, heart disease, high blood pressure are all diet-related health issues that cost this country more than 120 billion dollars each year," states First Lady Michelle Obama.

Another converging path... Dr. Esselstyn was beginning his career as a surgeon at the Cleveland Clinic

Dr. Caldwell Esselstyn began his career as a surgeon at the Cleveland Clinic. He and his colleagues were removing parts of the body that were not working properly... gallbladders, hernias, breast cancers, and coronary arteries.

In 1967, Esselstyn's colleague at the Cleveland Clinic, Dr. René Favaloro, removed a vein from a patient's leg and stitched it onto the heart's blocked coronary artery to allow the blood to flow around or bypass the blockage. Today 500,000 coronary bypass surgeries at $100,000 each are performed every year for a total of $50 billion!

By 1978, Esselstyn, who was the Chairman of the Breast Cancer Task Force at the Cleveland Clinic, was beginning to doubt the medical strategy he had been using. "No matter how many of these operations I was doing for women who had breast cancer, I wasn't doing one single thing for the next unsuspecting victim," lamented Esselstyn. There must be a better way to maintain our health.

Esselstyn began doing global research on cancer

When Esselstyn started doing research, the results were shocking. The chances of a woman getting breast cancer in Kenya were 82 times lower than in the U.S. In Japan in 1958 there were only 18 autopsy-proven deaths from prostate cancer. In the U.S. where the population was only twice that of Japan's and you might expect 40 or 50 deaths to occur, but no, there were more than 14,000. *Yes, 18 versus 14,000!* The risk of heart disease in rural China was 12 times lower than in the U.S. in the 1970s. In Papua, New Guinea heart disease was rarely seen. Why?

They did not eat a Western Diet. They did not consume animal products. No milk. No meat.

Then Esselstyn discovered some surprising historical data. "A study like this would have been impossible to do... take milk and meat away from a whole country's people. But there 'the study' was and the results were powerful."

During World War II Norway had little or no milk or meat. What happened to their health as result?

When World War II began, the Germans confiscated the animals and livestock for their troops, so the Norwegian people were forced to eat primarily plant-based foods. And what was the result? Deaths from cancer fell sharply, says Esselstyn.

When the war was over and the Norwegians started eating meat and dairy again, the heart attack rate jumped right back up to where it was pre-war. "It's such an absolutely powerful lesson," says Esselstyn, "but we didn't get it."

Whoa! Before you rush to your refrigerator to toss out your beef, chicken and fish, there may be more to the story

Yes, the Norwegian story was a powerful lesson but a powerful lesson in what? In the reduction of meat and cancer? Or the impact of eating more fish, less sugar, and potatoes instead of wheat? Or the ingenuity of people? Let's take a look.

David and Goliath... but in this case David is Denise

Denise Minger, 23, stepped up to reanalyze the data published by Campbell. As researchers know all too well, once your results are published, and in this case Campbell's statistical raw data was also published, other researchers will re-think, re-examine and come to their own conclusions. The beauty of data is, it talks and talks louder than titles and reputations. So there's a face off going on between Denise and the two Goliaths. Of course, there are other researchers weighing in on this as well.

Minger writes, "For the record, I'm not dissecting this movie because I think everything in it is terrible. Quite the opposite, in fact. I believe the 'plant-based diet doctors' got a lot of things right, and a diet of whole, unprocessed plant foods (i.e., Real Food) *can* bring tremendous health improvements for people who were formerly eating a low-nutrient, high-crap diet. Especially short term. But I also believe this type of diet achieves some of its success by accident, and that the perks of eliminating processed junk are inaccurately attributed to eliminating all animal foods. So the goal of this critique is to shed light on the areas where the plant-based science is a little, um, wilted."[37]

Minger takes Campbell's statements one by one at great length with backup statistics and graphs in her article *The China Study: Fact or Fallacy?*[38] To give you a feel for it, we will mention a few. For example, Minger points out that in the 20%/5% cancer on and off statement Campbell substituted the words *animal protein in place of *casein or milk protein.* (I marked them with asterisks as noted.)

She questions the assumption that isolated casein in rat studies necessarily behaves the same way other animal protein sources and combinations act in the body.

Minger writes, "As ample literature indicates other forms of animal protein—particularly whey, another component of milk—may have strong anti-cancer properties. Some studies have examined the effect of whey and casein, side-by-side, on tumor growth and cancer, showing in nearly all cases that these two proteins have dramatically different effects on tumorigenesis (with whey being protective).

A study Campbell helped conduct with one of his grad students in the 1980s showed that the cancer-promoting abilities of fish protein depended on what type of fat is consumed alongside it. The relationship between animal protein and cancer is obviously complex, situationally-dependent, and bound with other substances found in animal foods—making it impossible to extrapolate anything universal from a link between isolated casein and cancer."

She also notes that Campbell never mentions these Indian researchers actually published this paper as part of a two-paper set, one showing that low-casein diets make aflatoxin much more acutely toxic to rats." And the other showing rats on low protein diets exposed to aflatoxin experience more actual liver damage and more deaths than rats on high-protein diets. In all, 30 rats on the high-protein diet and 12 on the low-protein diet survived for more than a year."[39]

The China Study... what part did wheat play?

I was unaware of Denise Minger until I saw that Davis had devoted six pages to her reanalysis of The China Study data in his book, *Wheat Belly*.[40] Minger pointed something Davis felt was worthy of note about the effects of wheat.

"Although wheat gets nary a mention in the China Study chapter, Campbell actually found that wheat consumption—in stark contrast to rice—was powerfully associated with higher insulin levels, higher triglycerides, coronary heart disease, stroke and hypertensive heart disease within the China Study data—far more so than any other food."[41]

Campbell has responded to Minger's challenges and you can read his responses online.[42] Minger's challenges and Campbell's rebuttals noted, let's return to *Forks and Knives*.

How about Esselstyn's assumption that the Norwegians were eating a plant-based diet during the war years?

No, according to Norwegian records of the time, instead of meat and dairy they were eating fish, fish roe and potatoes. A 200% increase in fish consumption! Sugar consumption was cut in half and butter and margarine intake was reduced significantly as well. Maybe these factors could account for the drop in the heart attack rate.[43]

The Norwegian home economics institutes focused the population on "how to exploit local resources from the sea and wild plants by experimenting with uncommon ingredients such as wild sea birds (including sea gull) and wild plants including moss."[44] "Apparently, a popular dessert was also "herring roe bread pudding," made mostly from fish eggs and potatoes*:

Recipe for herring roe bread pudding

350 g. herring roe; 1 tbs potato flour; 1 tbs bread flour; 5 tbs breadcrumbs; 4 boiled potatoes; 4 dl. milk; 1 tsp currants (made of dried blueberries); 2-3 tbs sugar; essence of almond; Served with sweet red sauce (*saftsaus*)."[45]

The Norwegian war experience, *Forks Over Knives*, *The China Study*... it seems the jury is still out on the animal versus plant protein debate as we seek to lose weight and regain our health. We are just beginning to understand the complexities of God's foods.

Other food approaches... Pritikin, Paleo, Blood Type and Chinese Medicine

Diets are like a pan of water sloshing. Back and forth. High fat, low fat. High vegetable, high animal. Back and forth. Slosh, slosh.

The Pritikin Diet is now The Calorie Density Solution

Most of us have heard of the Pritikin Diet: a low-fat though not vegetarian diet largely based on vegetables, grains, and fruits. Fat consumption is held to 10%.

Since 1976, more than 70,000 people have spent time at the Pritikin Longevity Centers learning how to eat and prepare low-fat meals and snacks as well as how to incorporate exercise and stress-reduction techniques in their lives. Originally Nathan Pritikin designed the program to lower cholesterol and help diabetics normalize their blood sugar without taking insulin. And people lost weight in the process.

The Calorie Density Solution

Now Nathan's son, Robert Pritikin, has updated the program, presenting what he calls *The Calorie Density Solution*.

He says the issue is not calories but how many calories are in a given amount of food... calorie density. A pound of broccoli has 130 calories but a pound of chocolate chip cookies has 2,140 calories. A large number of calories in a small amount of food like cookies is calorie dense.

"Choosing foods that have low calorie density, like apples and oatmeal, will allow you to eat until you are full and never force you to limit portion size or go hungry to lose weight." The higher the calorie density of a food, the more likely it is to cause weight gain. Why? Because you will need to eat more calories to feel full.[46]

Five hundred calories of plant food stretches your stomach full. 500 calories of processed food stretches your stomach half full. 500 calories of oil produces almost no fullness at all. So then you want to eat more and more and more... remember the former head of the FDA who was dumpster diving to discover the ingredients in the Chili's Southwestern Eggrolls and Boneless Shanghai Wings he was addicted to?

Your satiation mechanisms, the stretch receptors and density receptors in your stomach wall, were designed to work with *whole foods*, not today's high calorie, low density processed foods. More mass, more full. Broccoli and sweet potatoes and your satiation receptors respond... ding, ding, ding, you're full. Stop eating.

Remember our old friends Ghrelin and Leptin

> *Ghrelin is the hormone that tells you start eating.*
> *Leptin is the hormone that tells you stop eating.*

Ghrelin is also the hormone that makes you likely to gain weight when you're sleep deprived. Lack of sleep raises your ghrelin levels and tells you to *start eating*.

Hunger and fullness are regulated by several feedback mechanisms. One signal comes from your stomach wall when it stretches to contain the meal you are eating. Nerve stretch receptors signal the brain (read in robot voice) "Your stomach is expanding. Begin to stop eating." At the same time, ghrelin levels start to decrease. The result, more impulses reach your brain that say "stop eating" than "start eating."

After you start eating, it takes *about 20 minutes* for the message to "stop eating" to reach your brain, says registered dietitian Joanne V. Lichten, Ph.D., author of *Dining Lean - How to Eat Healthy When You're Not at Home*. *If you are a speed eater, you may want to slow down* so you won't overeat before that signal ever reaches your brain.

Lichten also suggests that you stand up during your meal to sense how your stomach feels. If you feel comfortable but not over-full, then you've eaten enough. This will help you avoid realizing from the bloated feeling in your stomach, that you've over eaten when you stand up and push your chair back.

The "you've eaten" hormone

Cholecystokinin is a hormone produced by your digestive system that tells your brain "you've eaten." The more you eat, the more Cholecystokinin is released. When you diet and reduce food intake, your stomach cuts back on the amount of "you've-eaten-hormone" signaling you to eat more and go off your diet. Eating lots of fiber will help short circuit this built-in survival mechanism.

To avoid children's weight issues... take their plate away

If you want kids to maintain a healthy weight, the American Dietetic Association advises you *not to encourage them to clean their plates but instead to watch for signs of fullness*, such as restlessness at the table or playing with their food. When you see these signals, take their plate away or let your child leave the table. This approach will help prevent food aversion and overeating.[47]

Reminding you a second time... protein tames hunger pangs

In a new study in the *Journal of Clinical Endocrinology and Metabolism*, researchers found high-fat foods, like fast foods, raised ghrelin levels and increased hunger. Eating carbohydrates made people even hungrier. Only *proteins* lowered ghrelin levels substantially and helped tame hunger pangs. No doubt that's why early man was so eager to find meat... something to keep in mind when you want to feel full.

Pre-agricultural eating from 10,000 years ago

Dr. Loren Cordain, a professor at Colorado State University and the author of *The Paleo Diet*, gives us a sneak peek back in time... to the Old Stone Age when men and women were hunting, gathering and fishing their food. There was no refrigeration so they ate whatever they found.

What was available to them as they wandered? Wild meat, wild plants, eggs, roots, vegetables, nuts, berries, seeds, legumes, small wild melons, fish or an occasional tortoise. But there were no well-stocked grocery stores in the Old Stone Age so these foods were only available seasonally, by skill, luck or chance.

These are the foods we were genetically adapted to eat, but they are not the foods we are eating today. The meat they ate wasn't the same meat we eat today either. It was wild. It was fresh. It was lean... yes, fatter in summer and leaner in winter but even at its fattest it was still leaner than the meat we eat. Today 99% of our livestock is fed grain year round, raised on feedlots so fat levels are kept high and stable. And the quantities of meat we eat are far greater too.

What didn't Paleo man eat? No salt, no sugar, no dairy. Cordain says, try catching a hairy wild animal and milking it! Quite a picture!

Four generations ago, processed foods started replacing real foods

Today 70% of calories of the typical American diet come from processed foods... 25% of our calories come from *refined grains...* breads, cereal, rice and pasta. 20% of calories come from *refined sugars* including High Fructose Corn Syrup. Keep in mind, until the

Industrial Revolution began 200 years ago, sugar was a luxury only kings could afford. 17% of our calories come from refined oils, 16% from feedlot meats. 10% from dairy and then there is added salt and alcohol.

Of course there were no Cokes, fries, hot dogs and burgers. These foods did not exist in the Old Stone Age. Four generations ago these new and improved shelf-life foods began displacing real foods. And there has been a tremendous cost to our health ever since. "The genome has not been able to adapt," says Cordain.

In his book, *The Paleo Diet*, Cordain lays out a nutrition program based on eating foods we were genetically designed to eat... lean meats, fish and other foods that made up the diet of our Paleolithic ancestors.[4849]

For Dr. D'Adamo vegetable versus animal food comes down to Blood Type

I was a vegetarian for decades but at about age 50, that lifestyle or food-style no longer worked for me. I started exploring other diet possibilities and stumbled up Dr. Peter D'Adamo's book *Eat Right 4 your Type*. As I read about O types, I suddenly heard myself saying, That's me! And I kept reading.

Losing weight may depend on your blood type

A single drop of your blood is as unique as your fingerprint. Foods and supplements contain lectins which, *depending on your blood type,* interact differently with your cells. *Nutrients good for one type may be harmful to another.*

"*Your blood type* is a more reliable measure of your identity than race, culture, or geography. It *is a genetic blue-print for who you are... a guide to how you can live most healthfully.* The key to the significance of blood type can be found in the story of human evolution: Type O is the oldest; Type A evolved with agrarian society; Type B emerged as humans migrated north and into colder, harsher territories; and Type AB was a thoroughly modern adaptation, a result of the intermingling of disparate groups. This evolutionary story relates directly to the dietary needs of each blood type today." writes Dr. D'Adamo in his book *Eat Right 4 Your Type.*

Type O... Back to Africa and those long treks to find meat

Type O was the blood type of the hunter-gatherers, early humans who went on long treks and made dangerous kills. Their diet was high in protein and fat with very few carbohydrates... occasional berries, fruits, insects, leaves, and roots found in season. Constant physical exercise and calorie deprivation made them lean and mean. Today "the success of the Type O Diet depends on consuming lean, chemical-free meats, poultry, and fish," says D'Adamo." *Dairy and grains don't suit the O type's digestive system.* These foods did not become staples until later in human evolution.[50]

Type A... fresh, pure, organic vegetables

Type As thrive on the vegetarian diets of their more evolved and more settled farmer ancestors. Type As need foods that are fresh, pure and organic. They are the opposite of Os. While animal foods speed up the metabolism of Os, *animal foods slow down the metabolism of As, leaving them feeling sluggish and tired* and storing that protein as fat. A types thrive on plant proteins. Like Os, A types do not tolerate dairy foods well. They can eat wheat in limited quantities but soy has the advantage of increasing their metabolism.

Type B... Meat, liver, eggs and low fat dairy

Type Bs are a bit schizophrenic, in some ways like O Types but in other ways quite different. The B blood type seems to have united differing peoples and cultures. *Type Bs tend to resist severe diseases like heart disease and cancer* and, even if they contract them, tend to survive. Though wheat gluten doesn't affect B types as severely as it affects Os, wheat mixed with corn, lentils, buckwheat, sesame and peanuts is just as damaging. *However, to lose weight, Type Bs need to avoid wheat.* Eating moderate amounts of dairy helps B types achieve metabolic balance. Meat, liver, eggs and low fat dairy products aid the B type's metabolism.

Type AB... Tofu, seafood and green vegetables

Type AB blood has been around for less than 1,000 years. Only 2-5% of the population has AB blood. In general, foods that are bad for As and Bs are also bad for ABs. This type is typically stronger and more active than the more sedentary A types. *ABs lack the stomach acid needed to metabolize meats* efficiently so they tend to be stored as fat. *Tofu, seafood and green vegetables aid metabolic efficiency.* Dairy and kelp enhance insulin production.

O... Oh my heavens, that's me

D'Adamo presents a complete manual for each type... foods that are beneficial and foods to avoid. Complete description of each type, menus and exercise suggestions.

I was amazed when I read my O-type profile in *Eat Right 4 Your Type*. The foods that I knew didn't agree with me were listed as Avoid Foods. The foods I had learned over a lifetime worked for me were listed as Beneficial. And it was fascinating to discover major health issues I had confronted were common to my type. Eating more Beneficial Foods has improved my digestion significantly. Eating for my blood type has affirmed what my inner knower had been trying to tell me all along, what friends and manufacturers had been urging me to ignore. A most basic truth... some foods and exercises work better for me than others. Better for my blood type and body.

D'Adamo's family were Type As. Young Peter's friends thought he and his family were weird. While they were pigging out on hot dogs, french fries, hamburgers and sodas, Peter and his family were chowing down on tofu, steamed vegetables and salads. Looks to me like Peter's Mom and Dad, Dr. James D'Adamo who first began the study of blood types, made a wise choice. A choice that effectively met their A type-family needs.[5152]

Which diets work best for your type?

"My patients often ask me about current diet plans that are in vogue. The latest are the high-protein diets. By severely limiting carbohydrates, high-protein diets force the burning of fats for energy and the production of ketones, which indicate a high rate of metabolic activity. It doesn't surprise me that the patients who tell me they have lost weight on high-protein diets are usually Type Os and Type Bs," remarks D'Adamo.

On the other hand he says the macrobiotic diet which includes vegetables, rice, whole grains, fruits, and soy, may be best suited for Type As provided they consume recommended grains and legumes.

"The bottom line: Anytime you see a new diet plan that claims to work the same way for everyone, be skeptical. The dynamics of weight loss are related to the changes your body makes when you follow your genetically tailored diet. Listen to your blood type," writes D'Adamo.

There's more to food. There's food as medicine

Susan's mother-in-law is Chinese and she has a different soup for each season as well as foods and herbs for every condition... congestion, fever or upset stomach. Roots in winter, raw fruits and vegetables in summer. Ginger and lotus root, dioscorea and astragalus. And, her food remedies work.

Somehow we have forgotten the medicinal element of food. If you take a minute or two to think back in your particular ethnic tradition, you will probably remember foods your grandparents used as medicine. I remember lots and lots of chicken soup!

Chinese Medicine... ageless wisdom

"A diet consisting mainly of raw fruits and vegetables cools not because these foods have been refrigerated, but because they promote loss of body heat and the secretion of fluid. For a person who is Cold, Damp, and depleted, this diet exaggerates *internal* climate, aggravating symptoms of chilliness, puffiness, phlegm, fullness, and fatigue. Similarly, a diet consisting of fried, broiled, fat-rich, and spicy foods warms since these foods have absorbed the heat of cooking and because they generate body heat and stimulate circulation. For a person who is Hot, Dry, and congested, these foods exacerbate existing problems such as nervousness, sweating, tension, pain, constipation, and thirst. The same salads and juicy fruits that undermine an already cool, moist person are therapeutic for someone who is hot and dry; and the warm stimulation of spicy, broiled, and enriching foods that congest one person strengthen another," write Harriet

Bienfield and Efrem Korngold in *Between Heaven and Earth: A Guide to Chinese Medicine.* [53]

"To the majority of Americans these considerations are alien. Our diet conforms more to the dictates and demands of the marketplace—we eat quick, easy, tasty meals and buy what advertising sells us. We've lost touch with what feels good or is good for us. We have a distorted relationship to food: starving ourselves to cast off unwanted weight and overeating as a substitute for real pleasure and satisfaction. To meet our demands for intense, constant productivity, we relentlessly overstimulate our bodies with high-protein, high-fat, high-sugar foods that have become associated with affluence and the good life."[54]

> He that takes medicine and neglects diet,
> wastes the skills of the physician.
> Ancient Chinese Proverb

Here are all 10 Diet Skills...

Diet Skill One: Success Filing... when your Success File is full, you feel Success-Full

Diet Skill Two: Updating... will your past suck you back? Or will your future pull you ahead?

Diet Skill Three: Shifting Gears... starting, accelerating and creating your own weight loss

Diet Skill Four: Hologramming... how to get what you want far more easily

Diet Skill Five: Switching... the Alchemy of Success, how to turn negatives into gold

Diet Skill Six: Codreaming or co-dreading... the difference between getting fat and getting thin

Diet Skill Seven: Finding experts... who are also codreamers

Diet Skill Eight: Shielding... raising your infant dream

Diet Skill Nine: Committing to outcome... instead of hanging on to familiar methods

Diet Skill Ten: Maintaining your health and balance, and our planet's

No one can stay on "a diet" forever, but you can make a foodstyle transformation whenever you choose. Forget about skill numbers.
Bottom line... use 'em when you need 'em!

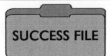

SUCCESS FILE

Time to Success File again...
Diet Skill Nine: Committing to Outcome

What outcomes are you committed to? Which old methods might you need to let go of to get there?

Do you have an upcoming event scheduled you want to feel slim and fit for? When is it? What are you planning to wear? And what are you doing to be able to wear it?

Who do you know who has an outcome in mind and needs your support? And who might be stuck in an old, familiar method?

Which diets do you think will work best for you? Which foods do you know are" medicine" for you? Chicken soup or grapes or ...?

Do you know what your blood type is? Have you explored which foods are beneficial to your type and which ones to avoid?

Do you do well on a plant-based diet or do you feel your body needs animal protein? Which diets have worked well for you and which haven't?

How does your body react to milk and cheese? To wheat and grain? To sugar and caffeine? What foods do you crave or feel addicted to? Is continuing to eat the foods you crave more important to you than your weight and health?

Turn to the back now and add as many more Successes as you can.

Diet Skill Ten: Maintaining your health and balance... and our planet's

Here we are, standing side by side as partners in exploration... food exploration. We know all 10 skills now as we head forward. We used to think about losing weight through the eyes of a particular diet. But let's look more broadly at what it will take to normalize your weight and regain your health. Not short term but long term. The 10th Diet skill takes us into a new realm... into 3rd gear exploration and discovery. A Grand Experiment.

A strange pair of problems... malnutrition and obesity

An odd combination, isn't it? How can we solve Earth's greatest problems... malnutrition and obesity... *and honor our environment at the same time?* How can we properly nourish not just ourselves but everyone on our planet? What are researchers discovering that you need to know, and share?

Losing weight and gaining health is a change you will be making for the rest of your life. One method will not be enough, or two or five or ten or even a hundred. As your life, body and environment change, you will need to be able to *sense* when a different approach is needed and be willing to modify even your most sacred routines.

Humans need change... change in foods, change in exercise, change in routines, change in people and change in focus. Stasis simply doesn't suit our God-given minds and bodies. We can't perceive anything clearly until it moves and changes, an animal, a

Time to help the next generation live healthy

When Bill Clinton was 13, he already weighed 185 pounds. When he was President we frequently saw him on TV chowing down on fast foods. When he was 58, he had his first heart attack and quadruple bypass.

Pastry chef Mesnier said when Clinton came to the White House he had a "scary" appetite. He could eat five or six pork chops and he loved desserts. "Mesnier recalls the episode of a strawberry cake he made one evening. Clinton devoured half of it all by himself, and the next morning he wanted more. No one could find the cake, says Mesnier who had a face-to-face with the distraught commander-in-chief. Clinton was pounding on the table and shouting, I want my cake."[55]

What tastes good may not be good for our bodies

No, what tastes good to us and the quantities that feel good to us may not be good for our bodies. And the changes we make, based on familiar tastes and habits, may not be enough either. Like it or not, ready or not, sometimes our bodies demand drastic action.

Clinton's first heart attack did not come on suddenly though it may have seemed that way to the public. *Jack Sprat He's Not* was the title of a 1992 *NPR News Blog* that revealed Clinton preferred foods that contained lots of fat: jalapeño cheeseburgers, chicken enchiladas, barbecue, cinnamon rolls and pies.[56]

For years Clinton had been overeating, and he had a family history of heart disease as well. What, you say? If Clinton knew he had a family history of heart disease, why didn't he make changes? Great question, but *unfortunately even the smartest of us doesn't always do the smart thing.*

Yes, the President had made attempts to diet over the years. In 1993, First Lady Hillary Clinton asked Dr. Dean Ornish to design a diet healthier than the high-fat French cuisine the White House chef had been serving. Ornish changed the menu to include soy burgers, stir-fry vegetables with tofu and salmon with vegetables. But that change in the White House food was not enough. Clinton was not always "eating at home." He was out and about campaigning and attending state dinners across America and around the world. By 1999 Clinton had put on an additional 18 pounds and plaque was building up in his coronary arteries.

Even though Clinton lowered his calorie and cholesterol intake, when he was in Haiti after their devastating 2010 earthquake, his heart problems resurfaced. This time he needed to have two stents (mesh tubes) inserted to open one of the veins from his quadruple bypass surgery. The vein had become, in Clinton's words, "pretty bent and ugly."

A few days after his surgery, Clinton met with Ornish who told him "that because of his genetics, moderate changes in diet and lifestyle weren't enough to keep his disease from progressing. However, our research showed that *more intensive changes actually reverse progression of heart disease in most people."*

Clinton finally committed to making drastic changes. "I essentially concluded that I had played Russian roulette" with my health. Today Clinton eats no meat, no dairy, no eggs, and almost no oil. His experts and codreamers are Drs. Ornish and Esselstyn. "All my blood tests are good, and my vital signs are good, and I feel good, and I also have, believe it or not, more energy," Clinton chuckled.[57] His latest goal is to get his weight down to 185, the weight he was when he was 13 years old!

Now Clinton doesn't *only* want to heal himself. The Clinton Foundation and the American Heart Association are working together to help 12,000 schools promote exercise and provide higher-quality lunches so today's kids won't have to face the same heart troubles he has."It's turning a ship around before it hits the iceberg, but I think we're beginning to turn it around," Clinton said.[58]

Whether Clinton's diet is the one you want to commit to or another diet seems to fit you better, it's time for drastic action. It's time to commit to change!

We are not just responsible for our weight and health but our children's weight and health as well. What we do not know ourselves and we do not do ourselves could affect their health for the rest of their lives. Remember, our children are watching. They have learned by our example. And they can be relearning by our example too!

Where is our children's health now? "Today's children may be the first generation to live shorter lives than their parents," reported CBS News.[59]

Our greatest weight challenge is our children... Pink Slime, GMOs and an extra China and India to feed

According to the American Heart Association in 2012, approximately 1 in 3 children ages 2–19 is overweight or obese... 32.1% of all boys and 31.3% of all girls.[60] According to the American Obesity Association, "45.9 percent of teens are at risk for developing weight-related health problems. Teens normally gain weight, but it is when weight gain increases beyond normal limits that teens become at risk for obesity."[61]

Unfortunately diabetes is worse in kids than adults

Heart disease is associated with obesity and so is diabetes. *And diabetes is particularly troublesome when it affects children.*

"Obesity and the form of diabetes linked to it are taking an even worse toll on America's youth than medical experts had realized. As obesity rates in children have climbed, so has the incidence of Type 2 diabetes, and a new study adds another worry: the disease progresses more rapidly in children than in adults and is harder to treat," writes Denise Grady in the *New York Times* April 29, 2012.[62]

Oral meds which work effectively for adults for many years only work for a year or two with kids. Then kids are forced to start giving themselves daily shots of insulin, and to figure out how much insulin to give.

I know how complicated it is to determine the right amount to inject. Remember my husband Albert has diabetes and I usually know when his blood sugar is too high or too low *before* he does. At that point, he's exhausted and fuzzy-headed and it's hard for him to make decisions. Blood sugar extremes play games with your head. If he gives himself too much insulin, he's shaking and blacking out. And if he gives himself too little, he's still in crisis. If he drinks too much juice or eats too much sugar, it makes it worse. He feels so desperate to get back to normal that he wants to down the whole bottle of juice but that would be a disaster. We always plan ahead and carry snacks to turn his blood sugar back in the right direction. If it's that hard for an adult, how much harder will it be for kids?

"It's frightening how severe this metabolic disease is in children," said Dr. David M. Nathan, director of the diabetes center at Massachusetts General Hospital. "It's really got a hold on them, and it's hard to turn around."[63]

Poorly-controlled diabetes significantly increases the risk of heart disease, eye problems, nerve damage, amputations and kidney failure, and *the longer a person has the disease, the greater the risk*. "I fear that these children are going to become sick earlier in their lives than we've ever seen before," Dr. Nathan said regretfully.

Key questions... what are your kids eating? And how much are they exercising?

Remember the key questions we asked you in the beginning of this book... what are you eating and how much of it are you eating? How much are you exercising and how much exercise do you need? These are the same key questions we need to be asking on behalf of our children.

You may know what they are eating a home but how about at school? Do your kids have gym class these days? How much are they exercising? Are they involved in after-school sports or leagues? Or, are they spending hours a day on the couch "exercising in the virtual world?"

Jamie Oliver's Food Revolution... school lunches

British Chef Jamie Oliver launched his TV show *Food Revolution* in the U.S. in 2010 to alert us to the poor quality of school lunches. This was a follow-up to a similar documentary series which first aired in England in 2005. After the show, in response to an online petition signed by a quarter of a million people, Prime Minister Tony Blair and his government banned certain junk foods from schools. Fried foods are limited to twice a week and soft drinks are no longer available.

When leading preventive cardiologist Dr. Arthur Agatston and his team began monitoring elementary students participating in an obesity-prevention program, their goal was "to show that good food was good for kids," says Agatston. "And that they would eat it."

Do your kids' lunches affect their grades? Yes, says the creator of the South Beach Diet

Agatston is best known for his *South Beach Diet*, which he originally devised as a way to help his cardiac and diabetes patients lose weight in order to prevent heart attacks and strokes. In 2004, he founded the Agatston Research Foundation, which now conducts and funds original research on diet, cardiac health, and disease prevention.

The two-year Healthier Options for Public Schoolchildren (HOPS) study found that "kids who ate nutritionally sound, high-quality breakfasts, lunches, and snacks — instead of the typical cafeteria food — not only had lower blood pressure and were less likely to be overweight, they also scored significantly better on standardized tests, especially in mathematics."[64]

Is Pink Slime in your kid's lunch?

One of Oliver's *Food Revolution* episodes left parents amazed and disgusted. He did a demonstration about Pink Slime. Yes, you read that right.[65]

Oliver stands next to a live cow which has maps drawn on its hide showing where various cuts are located... filets, steaks, chops and ribeyes... and their dollar value. Once the cuts have been made and the meat has been taken away, what is left is trimmings that butchers used to pay to have hauled away. "But what would you think if I told you that in America they have come up with a piece of technology to turn this into something that ends up in your school food? *Pink Slime is allowed in any school in America by the USDA!*" reveals Oliver.

What we don't know won't hurt us… or will it?

Here is how Pink Slime is made. They put these trimmings in a centrifuge and spin them to split the fat from the meat. Then they wash the meat bits in water and ammonia to kill e-coli and salmonella. (You probably have ammonia in the cabinet under your kitchen sink with a child lock on it. Why? Because it's poison.) Then they drain it and mince it. "So basically we are taking a product that would be sold in the cheapest form for dogs and, after we've processed it, we can give it to humans. Hamburgers, chilis, chopped steaks, tacos"… and to stretch ground beef they are allowed to add up to 15% of Pink Slime. You've just turned dog food into potentially *your* kids' food. And the USDA who is employed to protect you has made it legal to *not have to register* the ammonia on any label. They say it is a *process* not an *ingredient*.

How can you avoid feeding your family Pink Slime?

Oliver says, buy beef that comes from grass-fed cows at natural and organic grocery stores or at your local farmers' market. And have your butcher grind that meat for you while you watch.[66]

Jamie Oliver's *Food Revolution* won an Emmy Award in 2010 for Outstanding Reality Program but was pulled the second year after only a few episodes because of poor ratings. Guess there are some truths most people just don't want to know! But Oliver's work and his avid viewers have had an impact… whether manufacturers want to admit it or not.

McDonalds, Burger King and Taco Bell have eliminated it but 70% of U.S. ground beef products still contain it... and it's still in school lunches

"McDonald's confirmed that it has eliminated the use of ammonium hydroxide — an ingredient in fertilizers, household cleaners and some roll-your-own explosives —in its hamburgers. The company denied that its decision was influenced by a months-long campaign by celebrity chef Jamie Oliver to get ammonium-hydroxide-treated meats like chicken and beef out of the U.S. food supply. But it acknowledged this week that it had stopped using the unappetizing pink goo," according to NBCNews.com January 31, 2012. And Taco Bell and Burger King have followed suit.[67]

But hold on a minute. As of March 2012, Pink Slime, or *lean finely textured beef* (LFTB) as the USDA prefers to call it, is still admitted to be in 70% of ground beef products. Yes, everything from hamburger to chopped steak to processed and canned beef. *And it is still in school lunches.*[68] ABC News emailed the top 10 grocery chains in America. Only Publix, Costco, HEB and Whole Foods responded, saying they don't use Pink Slime. There was no response from the rest as of March 2012.

The food industry has *enormous* power over what is served in our schools and grocery stores. <u>And so do you when you speak up.</u> When you stop buying their products! And now, if you insist that schools stop serving Pink Slime in our kids' lunches and grocery stores stop selling it unless it's clearly labeled. Thanks to the internet and social media we can quickly broadcast information like this and find codreamers who will take action along us.

"The shared meal elevates eating from a mechanical process of fueling the body to a ritual of family and community, from the mere animal biology to an act of culture," writes Michael Pollan, author of *The Omnivore's Dilemma.*

Unlike L.A., Appleton's school lunch experiment was a resounding success

"Before Appleton, Wisconsin's high school replaced their cafeteria's processed foods with wholesome, nutritious food, the school was described as out-of-control. There were weapons violations, student disruptions, and a cop on duty full-time. After the change in school meals, the students were calm, focused, and orderly. There were no more weapons violations, and no suicides, expulsions, dropouts, or drug violations. The new diet and improved behavior has lasted for seven years, and now other schools are changing their meal programs with similar results," writes Jeffrey M. Smith, author of *Seeds of Deception.*[69]

Our kids are curious about what they are eating

Our kids are curious about the foods they are eating. And they are taking action to explore and experiment. Appleton students are conducting experiments which will probably affect their whole lives, and ours.

One group of students fed three mice in cage one the whole foods they were used to eating. But they fed the three mice in cage two "junk food that kids in other high schools eat every day." The behavior of the junk-food eating mice changed drastically. They destroyed their cardboard sleeping tubes and stayed awake all night and day. They no longer played together but they began fiercely fighting among themselves. Finally two mice killed the third and ate it.

What a shocking result from just a small change in food! After three months, the students shifted the surviving mice's diet back to whole foods, and *in about three weeks* they returned to normal.

GMO foods and unintended consequences

A student in Holland was interested in the effects of Genetically Modified (GM or GMO) foods. He fed one group of mice GMO corn and soy and the other non-GMO. The GMO-fed mice stopped playing together. When he tried to pick these usually-calm creatures up, they ran around in fear and tried to climb the walls. At the end of the experiment, one mouse in the GMO group was found dead in the cage.[70]

Shocking but maybe this study can shed some light on their reaction. A study in *Science* December 2002 concluded that "*food molecules act like hormones*, regulating body functioning and triggering cell division. The molecules can cause mental imbalances ranging from *attention-deficit and hyperactivity disorder to serious mental illness.*"[71]

Animals seem to be food-smarter than humans. Eyewitnesses across America have reported that cows, pigs, elk, deer, raccoons, squirrels, rats and mice avoided eating GMO food when they were given a choice.

Missing Monsanto files found... guess we weren't told the whole truth

For some reason, a side-by-side comparison between GMO and non-GMO soy was *not* included in a paper published by Monsanto in the *Journal of Nutrition* in 1996. When a medical writer found the missing data in the archives years later, it became clear why that comparison had been left out. "The GMO soy showed significantly lower levels of protein, a fatty acid, and phenylalanine, an essential amino acid. Also, toasted GMO soy meal contained nearly twice the amount of a lectin that may block the body's ability to assimilate other nutrients. Furthermore, the toasted GMO soy contained as much as seven times the amount of trypsin inhibitor. (This might explain the *50 percent jump in soy allergies* in the UK, just after GMO soy was introduced,)" says the Organic Consumers Association.[72]

Interestingly, the Appleton school lunch program was not designed to eliminate GMO products but because GMO foods are contained in processed foods, when processed foods were eliminated almost all GMO ingredients were too.

"Since children are three to four times more susceptible to allergies, changes in GMO food are likely to have a much larger impact on children. Thousands of schools around the world, particularly in Europe, have decided not to let their kids be used as guinea pigs," writes Smith. "They have banned GMO foods."

The Whole Foods Market chain is specifically committed to clearly labeling GMO ingredients so their shoppers can avoid these foods if they choose.[73]

What undiscovered life-sustaining compounds could change or disappear?

Science is just beginning to catch up with the inner workings of God's miraculous foods. In fact, we have just started to identify medicinal compounds they contain.

"Blueberries have compounds that boost neuron signals and help turn back on systems in the brain. In contrast, people with

Alzheimer's disease have weaker neuron signals. Eating blueberries and a diet rich in deep pigment from fruits and vegetables can boost the potency of neuron signals," says Dr. James Joseph of the USDA Human Nutrition and Research Center on Aging at Tufts University.[74]

Eating strawberries and blueberries before radiation helped rats experience fewer side effects and may also help humans. Further study is in process. The antioxidant in grape skins may fight cancer and reduce heart disease. When mice and rats ate blueberries they experienced fewer occurrences of Alzheimer's disease and arthritic inflammation.[75]

A quick review... from slow evolutionary changes to quick, short-sighted modifications

When did this all begin?

"The first tentative moves that got life out of the water and onto the land eons ago were apparently made by slimy green algae, scientists say, and coming ashore wasn't easy. Even though four distinct types of algae managed to come ashore, only one of them evolved enough complexity to eventually cover the land with vegetation, what we now call trees, shrubs, flowers, and grass," says National Geographic News.[76]

For eons we had been eating The Miracle Diet. We may not always have had enough food, but the foods we ate were whole. However during this century, for better or worse, man started modifying God's foods. Modified foods may look the same, but they don't work the same way in our bodies. We are just beginning to understand the health impacts these modifications are having.

Agro scientists used their emerging know-how to hybridize a "new wheat" which is easier to harvest, but which Davis has discovered is producing obesity, *Wheat Belly* and severe allergies. Unfortunately agro-scientists took their "new wheat" to market without animal or human testing. *Bottom line, they have been testing their "new wheat" on us.*

Even though hybridization lacks the precision of gene modification techniques, it still possesses the potential to inadvertently *turn genes on* or *off.* Remember, "genes are not Legos; they don't just snap into place. Gene insertion creates *unpredicted, irreversible changes,*" says Smith.

GMO soybeans may be linked to infant mortality and the inability to conceive. In a two-year study, after three generations, most of the GMO-soy fed hamsters lost the ability to reproduce. *Sadly, we don't know enough yet to know what these DNA changes will ultimately produce.*[77]

In the 1950s we made a sharp turn... from home-cooked, farm-raised foods to burgers, drive-ins, supermarkets and convenience items. And we started eating far more... twice as much meat, 20 times more dairy, 4 times more sugar and the illness rates from diabetes, cancer, heart disease and obesity soared.

With more people wanting more food, agricultural scientists went to work to enhance their color, texture, taste, nutrition, *and* to meet agro-business's need to bring foods to harvest quicker, easier and bug-free.

With Americans eating out, taking out and ordering in more and more, food producers started adding concentrated amounts of salt, fat, and sugars (The Addictive Mix) to our food. This is the combination former FDA head Kessler says is addicting our brains and our children's brains and compelling us to overeat these toxic foods.

Sadly this century's "scientific advances" have not made Americans healthier. Instead we have gotten fatter and sicker.

Another "New Wheat"… "Whiffy Wheat"

For better or worse, more changes are on the way. "The world's first GMO crop that has been deliberately engineered to emit a repellent-smelling substance against insect pests is now growing in a small patch of land in the Hertfordshire countryside (of England.) Scientists have created the "whiffy" wheat in an effort to combat aphid attacks," reports Steve Connor in *The Independent*, an English daily newspaper March 29, 2012.[78]

We are living in the midst of "A Grand Experiment"

Not only have we modified our foods but we have also modified our planet… without understanding the intricacies of how our world works any better than we have understood the intricacies of our foods.

We have made poorly thought-through, short-term decisions, paved over farmland, bulldozed and blacktopped roadways up and around mountains, through valleys and across plains. We have overfished our rivers and oceans, cut down trees and put up parking lots.

We cleared land to raise tobacco, cotton, rubber, cattle, corn or sugar, whichever was the cash crop of the day. We built factories whose smoke stacks are polluting our air. We stopped walking and started driving almost everywhere.

We have over-populated and defoliated once lush tropical areas so nothing grows on hills to hold back the soil, to keep the rain from digging deep furrows down their sides, leaving no plants or trees to create shade or release oxygen.

More cities, more people. Less farmland, fewer acres of forest and open land. Bulldozed, cleared, planted. Over planted. Over fertilized. Stripped.

We have diverted rivers leaving large areas of our planet's surface without water and irrigation so those areas are no longer farmable and life-sustaining. We have depleted our planet's soil, plants, foods and animals. *And we have depleted ourselves*.

Sharp turns in how we eat, how we plant and farm

On the farm we made sharp turns too... from seeds grown and stored by farmers to plant the next season, to seeds sold by GMO producers that have to be bought again next season. And these seeds require irrigation and are designed to be used with pesticides these same companies sell.

Here's another devastating unintended consequence. The 2011 documentary film *Bitter Seeds* states, "Every 30 minutes, a farmer commits suicide in India. For millennia, farmers in India had cultivated cotton with seeds they'd saved from their own plants. Hybrid seeds cannot be saved, so the farmers had to buy more seeds each year. In time, the hybrids required more costly pesticides, as well. Farmer suicides began in 1997, as many went into debt and couldn't make ends meet." They lost their land, their ability to support their families and finally their pride.[79]

The Green Revolution produced unintended consequences too

Yes, we are in the midst of "A Grand Experiment" here on Earth. And yes, we are getting smarter and more skillful as we progress, but what else have we done that is already affecting us, or is about to?

"Fifty years ago, when the world's population was around half what it is now, the answer to looming famines was "the green revolution" – a massive increase in the use of hybrid seeds and chemical fertilizers. It worked, but at a great ecological price. We grow nearly twice as much food as we did just a generation ago, but we use *three times as much water* from rivers and underground supplies," writes John Vidal of *The Observer* January 21, 2012. Here's another question: Is water our next global crisis?[80] Could this be another *crisis of our own making that will impact our children's lives?*

We've made mistakes but we're making advances too

Unfortunately it's always true. The more we practice, the better we get.

Lack of knowledge got us into this dilemma and increasing knowledge can bring us out of it... *if* we shift into 3rd gear exploration and discovery. *If* we codream and collaborate.

"The single greatest lesson the garden teaches is that our relationship to the planet need not be zero-sum, and that as long as the sun still shines and people still can plan and plant, think and do, we can, if we bother to try, find ways to provide for ourselves without diminishing the world," writes Pollan.

How else could we feed all Earth's people?

"The food choices we make have profound global effects. It takes *over 10 times* the amount of energy from fossil fuels to produce a calorie of animal-based food than it does to produce a calorie of plant food," reveals the movie *Forks over Knives*. "The world's cattle alone eat enough grain to feed 8.7 billion people, nearly 2 billion more than the population on Earth. With almost a billion malnourished people across the globe, redirecting even a portion of the grain used to fatten cattle could feed every hungry mouth on the planet."[81]

We usually think of plants as needing sun, water and soil but today food plants require a lot of petroleum energy too... the energy to transport them thousands of miles from the field to your store and your home. Most foods on your grocer's shelves have traveled an average of 1,500 miles! But some have journeyed far more. Grapes grown in Chile, transported by ship to California and shipped by truck to Iowa have traveled over 4,200 miles. A typical carrot has traveled 1,838 miles to reach your dinner plate.

Some studies argue that growing food only accounts for 21% of the energy required for many food products. Transportation (14%), processing (16%), packaging (7%), food retailing (4%), restaurants and caterers (7%) and home refrigeration and preparation (32%) account for the rest.

"Hawaiian pineapples are among the most carbon intensive foods, contributing about 40 pounds of CO_2 per pound of pineapple. That is about 10 times the next highest figure among the foods studied." Some agricultural scientists have proposed ecolabeling food based on CO_2 rankings.[82]

So, eat local as often as you can. Eat fresh foods instead of processed foods that have traveled from field to factory to store to you. As you know now, most Americans eat too much protein, about twice as much as is healthy[83] so start making up the difference with fresh fruits and vegetables. And remember, foods grown in your garden have never been on a truck, train or plane and are fresh and full of nutrients. Time and travel reduce vital nutrients. For example, fresh peas can lose up to 50 percent of their nutrients within a week of harvesting. Spinach stored at room temperature loses 50-90 percent of its vitamin C within 24 hours.[84]

Looking ahead to 2050... the food challenge is accelerating

"How can we feed the 2.5 billion more people – an extra China and India – likely to be alive in 2050? The UN says we will have to nearly double our food production and governments say we should adopt new technologies and avoid waste, but however you cut it, there are already one billion chronically hungry people.

Food, farm and water technologists will have to find new ways to grow more crops in places that until now were hard or impossible to farm. It may need a total rethink over how we use land and water. So enter a new generation of radical farmers, novel foods and bright ideas," writes Vidal.[85]

Orange sweet potatoes... saving the malnourished in Africa

For the huge population of under-nourished and malnourished Africa, the orange sweet potato may be the answer to a Vitamin A deficiency most common in children. This deficiency if severe can lead to blindness and premature death.

The orange sweet potato, the one we enjoy at Thanksgiving here in the U.S., is rich in beta-carotene which is a precursor to Vitamin A, and gives it its bright orange color. In Africa yellow and white sweet potatoes are more common but they do not contain enough beta-carotene to prevent these deficiencies. Only the orange sweet potato contains enough. This is a wonderful discovery. It will be just as easy to grow the orange beta-carotene-loaded ones, now that we know.[86]

New solutions, younger leaders

Other solutions like this will be found when we put our heads together... growing vegetables on rooftops, in community gardens, planting edible perennials instead of annuals, greening deserts and harvesting algae.... surely we don't need to wait for severe flood, drought or war to make food prices skyrocket and force us to consider other possibilities.[878889] And other solutions will be found when our kids put their heads together too. When their research comes to fruition or they decide to take action on their own.

They're bright. They're bold. They're explorers and innovators. They are our future.

16 year old Rami didn't wait until he was 58

Fortunately, unlike Clinton, 16 year old Rami didn't wait until he was 58. Or until he had coronary disease either. He took action early.

On June 27, 2011, Rami woke up saying, "Today is the day! I can't bear being fat anymore. I can't stand having the kids at school making fun of me."

Rami recalls that transformative moment clearly. He had started diets before so he knew what to do, but those had been false starts. This time Rami was sure he was going to become fit and lean. And he did!

"A couple of months before my 16th birthday, my family and I spent the day at the county fair. As we walked along, we passed a weight-guessing booth. If the man guessed correctly, you got nothing and he kept your money, but if he guessed wrong, you got a prize. That sounded good to me." The man guessed Rami weighed 260-something, but when Rami got on the scale the needle zoomed up and around to 303. "At first I thought, Oh great, I won the prize. But months later I realized the prize wasn't worth it."

Since 5th grade, Rami had been bigger than anyone else in his class. And, since 5th grade he had been taunted by his classmates. What were the kids saying to you, Rami, I asked? But he told me he couldn't repeat the words they had been using. They were awful words and they really hurt. At first he told his teachers what was going on, but all they did was say, "Stop making fun of Rami" and nothing changed. After that, the only person he talked to was his mom.

Rami's doctor was aware that he had been gaining weight little by little, but suddenly Rami's weight gain accelerated. "When I hit 9th grade I weighed 250 pounds. By 10th grade, I was at 286! I didn't care what I ate. I felt lazier and lazier. I didn't want to do anything." "Rami had terrible grooming habits in those days," his mom added, "but just look at him now. What a difference!"

Rami's weight was a touchy subject at home as well. His Mom got upset when family members made remarks at the dinner table... things like Rami, don't take another piece. Or, Rami, you don't need that. "Mom knew *if I was told not to eat* something I would eat it! (Remember, The Positive Command Brain.) Mom would take them aside and talk to them later. And she would find a private moment to lovingly deliver a supportive message to me."

Soon 16-year-old Rami's weight had soared to 310 pounds!

What were you eating? I asked

Quiet for a moment, Rami began, "My mom always kept a very healthy household, but when I went to the store I would sneak candy." How often did you go? Pretty often. Whenever Mom needed something I volunteered. How about junk food? I asked. Rami said No, they didn't eat fast food and never drank sodas at home either, and his mother nodded agreement.

But weighing 310 at age 16 was certainly *not usual*! So what was really going on here? Why was his weight gain so rapid and so steep?

Then his mom said, "Rami was eating *good stuff* but eating far too much of it." If anyone at the table took another helping, he wanted another helping too. And he shoveled it onto his plate. Rami's grandparents lived with his family that year. "Poppy ate very slowly, but I ate like a vacuum cleaner. He was always talking to me about food. He wants me to be healthy and still calls me every day."

But overeating at home didn't seem to explain Rami's accelerating weight gain either. So Susan and I kept asking questions. Rami's story still wasn't adding up... calorie wise and weight-wise.

I stopped at that point and asked Rami if I could read him a story... Loretta's story... and he nodded an enthusiastic YES. I read him the part about what John's mother was eating... two to three large bottles of Coke, a half dozen eggs, half a loaf of bread and two pieces of apple pie with ice cream... for breakfast.

Suddenly the flood gates of his memory opened wide

Rami wasn't just taking extra helpings, he was eating more than 3,000 calories for breakfast... 10 pancakes, 6 waffles or 6 huge slabs of French toast topped with butter and lots of maple syrup or chocolate syrup. Which one? I asked. Rami smiled, "Both of them. And lots and lots of milk. If Mom gave me fat free milk I'd complain."

It was like something turned in Rami's head and a door opened. Loretta's story held the key. Suddenly the picture became clearer. And then there was lunch.

Rami bought his lunch at school. What did he eat? Every day he ate 2 large slices of pizza (1 slice of Papa John's 14" Cheese Pizza, the brand they serve in his school, contains 304 calories) and three or four 6"cookies (at least 250 calories each). Plus 2 small bottles of Gatorade (90 calories each.) And, twice a day he would visit the vending machines in his school to buy Pop Tarts (219 calories for two) and an ice cream sandwich (180 calories)... and that's after those 10 pancakes (175 calories each) or 6 waffles, and two syrups (maple and chocolate) for breakfast.[90]

Rami, did you bring your lunch from home in elementary school? "No, I bought it at school then also. And those lunches were *no healthier*. We had pizza there too, or noodles with cheese on top, or two cheese sandwiches, plus 1 milk box and 1 juice box. But I never drank just one. I would collect 2-3 additional milks and juices. Plus we had dessert."

Every Saturday Rami went to the movies and woofed down two popcorns (with no butter) and, then thirsty, washed it down with Cherry Coke and free refills (140 calories per 8 oz which doesn't begin to fill the 54 oz cup size they sell.) And Rami is just one of thousands of teens who does this each weekend![91]

The Addictive Mix... fat, salt and sugar.
Rami was getting his junk food at school... and the movies

No, Rami wasn't eating fast food at home. He was eating it at school and at the movies. As you read on, keep this in mind. One medium popcorn *without butter* contains 11-16 cups (depending on which theater you're in), 650-900 calories and 43-60 grams of fat. You probably thought Rami's popcorn wasn't too bad because he didn't add butter. If he had, the calories would increase to 910-1220 calories and 71-97 grams of fat. That's more fat than in 6 McDonald cheeseburgers! And, depending on the type of oil used during popping, much of that fat is saturated fat which raises LDL cholesterol (the cholesterol that clogged up Bill Clinton's coronary arteries.)

But Rami didn't order a medium popcorn. He ordered one large *and got free refills*. A large popcorn at AMC Theatres has about 16 cups of popcorn and 1,000 calories, while a large at Regal Entertainment Group contains 20 cups and 1,200 calories, *and that's without butter. So two large popcorns were over 2,000 calories! And he may have had a third for free...* but like the prize he won for having his weight guessed wrong, those second, third or fourth free popcorns and cokes didn't turn out to be worth it in the end.[92]

Movie popcorn contains high amounts of saturated fat because most theaters use coconut oil or butter to pop it. According to the American Heart Association, the daily recommended intake of saturated fat is about 16 gm. A large popcorn from theaters that use coconut oil, including AMC and Regal, has about 60 gm of fat, *almost four times the daily recommended amount*. And lots of sodium too, about 1,400 gm in 16-20 cups. Remember the recommended amount of sodium is 1,250-2,300 gm a day![93]

At 16 Rami put *himself* on a diet and lost 100 pounds

"I cut out carbs and sugars, no corn or nuts, only salads with tomatoes and a couple of thick slices of turkey or a fish filet like tilapia. I cut my calories from over 6,000 to less than 2,000 a day. I was committed."

That summer Rami worked at a summer camp for 5-year-olds. My days were crazy. "The kids were climbing all over me. I took them on field trips, played with them on the jungle gym, threw balls and swam." Rami felt like a sheepherder trying to get the kids where they needed to go on time.

"One boy was the wildest in camp. He was sweet but he just didn't listen. He was finally starting to listen near the end of the summer but then camp was over. "He called me Froggy. I have no idea why. When I saw him later he remembered me by that name. Running around with five-year olds wasn't enough activity for me so I started going to the gym and walking or running two hours each day as well."

Rami has a sports mentality. You can't quit till it's over

One day Rami headed out for a run and it started raining. "I was clear that a little moisture wasn't going to stop me. I'm just going to run in the rain. It was nice exercising outdoors and soon, rain or shine, I was running 8 miles a day."

Rami, did you ever get tired, really tired? "Yes, there were days I woke up tired, but I have a sports mentality. You can't quit till it's over. I got up, got dressed and got going anyway. Nothing stopped me. I started my diet June 27 and toward the end of summer I had lost 48 pounds.

I was obsessed at that point. School was starting soon. What would the kids say to me this year? I was afraid that I was eating too many calories but I wasn't. I just didn't want to go back to my old ways. I actually lost another 12 pounds so when I went back to school I weighed 60 pounds less than when school had ended in June!

When I started 11th grade, everyone noticed my weight loss. Some kids were shocked and didn't even recognize me! It felt good to be noticed *positively* for a change. I even got my first kiss."

"Now instead of buying lunch at school, I bring it from home every day. A large salad with 1 small chicken breast or 2 fish filets. I made sure all the food in our house was healthy. Everyone else was getting mad at me. I just kept saying *but it's healthy*. My "skinny" little brother kept saying *but I like my junk*. By Thanksgiving I had lost 78 pounds!"

From 44 pants, I was down to 34

That fall Rami started football, but football didn't help him lose more weight. As he gained muscle, he actually gained weight. But he was getting stronger and tighter. "After practice, I was still doing two hours of running or walking."

"By February 13th, I had lost 100 pounds! From 310 to 210. Everyone was amazed! I was healthier. I was slimmer. I was stronger. And I was happier."

Guess what happened next... Rami's coach told him he needed to *gain* weight

Then Rami confronted an ironic twist. In February, "my coach said if you want to be able to take down guys 300 pounds or heavier, you will have to *gain* weight!" He told Rami he was the perfect weight for a linebacker, but he wasn't fast enough. "So I was stuck on the offensive or defensive line. I was disappointed at first but now I really love playing those positions. And I'm moving up the ranks."

Protein before, during and after work out

"Protein shakes ½ hour before and after exercising, and a protein bar while I was working out. I gained 18 pounds, but it wasn't fat I gained. It was muscle and that weight didn't add a single inch to my waist. Same pants size... still a 34."

When you're fat you don't realize you're fat, remembers Rami

"Since losing weight everything is easier, breathing, running, climbing stairs *and* meeting new friends. My old friends and I texted once in a while and hung out a little but we were all pretty inactive.

Since I lost weight, I have a new group of active, athletic best-friends, one of them is ranked 26th in Florida in tennis. Like me, they go to the gym every day. We're all athletic, active and exercising outside, not just playing video games and hanging out inside.

After losing 100 pounds and building muscle last year, I'm easing off a little, weighing myself every two weeks at the gym or on the Toledo scale at Publix. Since football muscle-building, I'm up to 231 and this is my baseline now.

I eat 2,000 calories a day and, given the calories I burn in football workouts plus running and my high percent of lean muscle, I know I'll stay trim. I am enjoying my new awareness of food and exercise. And my confidence is way up. I enjoy talking to girls... a lot of girls like me now. I am not embarrassed about my body. I go to the beach more often and I'm all around more open. I go to parties. I spend all my money on clothes. I really like looking my best."

Susan and I met Rami just as we were finishing this book, and we felt his story was one we needed to share with you. A 16 year old who "got it on his own" and he, unlike Clinton, did something drastic before his heart or his health forced him to take action. Now that Rami has lost 100 pounds, his real challenge begins. What will he need to change in his thinking and behavior *to maintain his weight loss long term*?

Like me, Rami immediately asked Susan what the 10 success skills are and how they work, and he's already reading this book to find out. He said he knows they will help with the rest of his life... including school and girls!

It's time to update your outcome

Rami, that "you can't quit till it's over" thinking contains a potential trap! Till what's over? Till you've lost 100 pounds? Then what? Will you slip back into old ways? Or will update your outcome *to maintaining a healthy weight for the rest of your life*? Then hopefully, because of your example, your children will maintain a healthy weight throughout their lives too. Rami, I know you're not thinking about that *yet*, but someday you will.

Obesity... the pandemic of our day

We are living amidst the greatest pandemic in human history... obesity and its profound health impact... diabetes, heart disease, high blood pressure and cancer to name a few. It directly affects each of us. We all see people we care about getting fatter and more inactive, more unhealthy and diseased, just as I saw my Dad dying slowly, toe-by-toe, day-by-day from diabetes.

Standing side by side and codreaming

Our multibillion dollar corporations employ millions of people and pay hundreds of billions of dollars in taxes. They are the delivery system of our food and healthcare. They are the backbone of our communities and economy.

We urge these corporations to look through a new set of lenses... how can you help people everywhere lose weight and gain health? How can *we all profit*, health-wise and money-wise, at the same time?

Examples of companies "looking through healthy lenses" are Whole Foods which is presenting a cornucopia of beautiful, healthy, natural foods. And, Costco which is providing consumers with more organic products at reasonable prices. And Walmart and Target, Publix and Krogers who are expanding their health food offerings. And more and more restaurants are providing Nutritional Labels. And offering gluten free menus... like P. F. Chang's, Chipotle and Panera Bread. And fresh organic menus, like *Michael's Genuine* in Miami. More fresh juice bars and smoothies. And, like Appleton, Wisconsin, more schools are not only serving healthy, whole food lunches but they are raising our children's awareness so they can make healthy choices at home, at school and the movies. What other companies can you recommend?

We also foresee... more and more businesses that will offer reasonably-priced, local, fresh foods and vegetables. Healthy food chains that serve organic grilled chicken, beef and vegetables. Local governments that provide outlets for farmers to sell their produce and provide space and mulch for community gardens. Weekly co-ops that buy fresh and local in bulk. And, the federal government providing more subsidies and insurance support for farmers who grow fruits and vegetables not just commodity crops like corn and soybeans.[94]

Yoga studios are popping up all over. Gyms are on almost every city corner. Acupuncture and Chinese medicine is rapidly gaining popularity. And the Slow Food movement is slowly gathering momentum. What else do you see on the horizon?

Enough is enough! Today is the day!

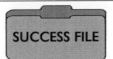

SUCCESS FILE

Time to Success File again...
Diet Skill Ten: Maintaining your health and balance...
and our planet's

Like Rami, when did you decide that enough is enough? Do you remember the day? What are doing now to rebalance your life? What changes have you made? What foods are you eating? What exercises are you doing? How have you altered your schedule?

Has your body been trying to tell you something? An ache, a pain, indigestion, high or low energy? Is diabetes or heart disease in your family? Who is your expert? Have you reached out?

Are the children in your family overweight? Do your kids take their lunch to school or buy it there? What do they eat, really? Pizza, dessert or fresh meats, vegetables and grains?

Do you know whether the ground meat you buy has Pink Slime in it? Or whether any foods you buy or eat have GMO ingredients?

Have you added more whole foods to your diet? How often do you eat out and where? Have you cut back on processed and fast foods? Do you have a garden or local food source?

What are you doing to rebalance our planet? Do you volunteer, write a newsletter or blog? Talk to school kids or groups? What organizations are you codreaming with, and which ones are codreaming with you? How are you making a difference?

You are invited to visit us at codreamsuccess.com

Join our Codreaming community. Share your success stories and solutions with us all. Tell us what you have learned and discovered about losing weight and gaining health. About specific foods and products. And, by all means, share your before and after pictures with us too!

When you sign up for our newsletter, *The Miracle Diet Update*, on our website, you will receive your Success File and Failure File as a gift so you can print and use them to update your life and build the self-confidence you need to do whatever you desire!

Like us on facebook. Follow us on twitter and Pinterest.

All best wishes! We hope to hear from you soon.

Susan Ford Collins and Rabbi Celso Cukierkorn

Other books to read by
Susan Ford Collins and Rabbi Celso Cukierkorn

The Joy of Success: 10 Essential Skills for Getting the Success YOU Want, **Susan Ford Collins**

"I have been reading books on success for over 30 years. This is one of the most sophisticated and useful ones I have ever read. I highly recommend it." **Jack Canfield, *Chicken Soup for the Soul***

Our Children Are Watching: 10 Skills for Leading the Next Generation to Success, **Susan Ford Collins**

"This may just be one of the most important books you will ever read in your life, important for you and for your children. A positively stunning book, *Our Children Are Watching* captured both my heart and my mind." **Chinaberry Book Service**

Shifting Gears: How YOU Can Succeed and Lead in the NEW Workplace, **Susan Ford Collins and Richard Israel**

"From our early beginnings we learn to 'shift gears' to survive. Finally, Susan Ford Collins and Richard Israel have put together a book all present and future business executives should make required reading." George A. Naddaff, **Founder, Boston Market**

$ecrets of Jewish Wealth Revealed: A Roadmap to Financial Prosperity, **Rabbi Celso Cukierkorn**

"This book provides a simple blueprint for daily financial discipline and shows us that with time, effort and a good plan, every dream is a possibility." Shaun Ince, **BMO Capital Markets**

Acknowledgments

There are so many people to thank! We are most grateful to all of you who codreamed this project with us and contributed your time and energy. Many people spent many hours reading *The Miracle Diet* out loud to us. We wanted to make sure that what we had in mind was actually written on these pages. Our readers questions, stumbles and misreads helped us fill in gaps and rearrange words and sentences to hopefully make your reading experience easier and smoother. And whenever we got tired, their energy kept us going!

Thanks to Dr. William Davis, author of *Wheat Belly,* for his clarifying input and guidance. Thanks to Alan Chaset for his legal support and to Ronald Montero for his marketing input.

Thanks to those of you who sat and read out loud to us!

We were fortunate to have had many people volunteer to read *The Miracle Diet out loud to us*. Many thanks to you all!

To Chris Morales, special thanks for your Wednesday afternoon full-volume radio announcer two-hour reads! Thanks to Penelope Friedland, Lynn Fish, Jesse Cukierkorn, Stacey Mosher, Bob Collins, Raquel Kopetman, Michael McCormick, Marilyn Rubin, Kristina Vecsesi, Fran Ford, Dylan Rosenberg, Cathy Rosenberg, Margaret Chaneles and Dmitry Zhitov. And many thanks to our cover designer Sharon Huff and our tech guru Albert Mah!

And bravo to our story tellers!

Thanks to those of you who shared your stories of weight loss and health gain with us and who answered our repeated queries for more and more and more detail. When our readers share how your stories inspired them in moments of doubt and resistance, we will be sure to pass on their comments to you!

Sources: Endnotes

[1] http://health.howstuffworks.com/wellness/food-nutrition/natural-foods/natural-weight-loss-food-mangoes-ga.htm

[2] http://en.wikipedia.org/wiki/Menachem_Mendel_of_Kotzk

[3] http://www.center4research.org/2011/08/a-guide-to-cholesterol-medication/

[4] http://www.reuters.com/article/2010/09/28/us-suicide-surgery-idUSTRE68R5FM20100928

[5] http://blogs.webmd.com/pamela-peeke-md/2011/05/its-baaack-weight-gain-after-lipo.html

[6] http://en.wikisource.org/wiki/The_Travels_of_Marco_Polo/Book_1/Chapter_28

[7] www.cdc.gov/salt/

[8] http://www.heart.org/HEARTORG/GettingHealthy/NutritionCenter/HealthyDietGoals/Sodium-Salt-or-Sodium-Chloride_UCM_303290_Article.jsp

[9] http://tuftshealthletter.com/ShowArticle.aspx?rowId=790

[10] http://wiki.answers.com/Q/How_much_sodium_in_one_teaspoon_salt

[11] http://www.acaloriecounter.com/food-labels.php

[12] Zinczenko and Goulding, *Grill This, Not That,* New York: Rodale, 2012

[13] http://www.diabeteshealth.com/read/1999/11/01/1700/do-i-subtract-fiber-from-carbohydrates/

[14] http://gmo-awareness.com/avoid-list/gmo-sodas/

[15] http://www.mendosa.com/gilists.htm

[16] Dr. William Davis, *Wheat Belly.* New York: Rodale, 2011.

[17] http://www.health.harvard.edu/newsweek/Glycemic_index_and_glycemic_load_for_100_foods.htm

[18] http://marshallbrain.com/science/sugar-in-soda.htm

[19] http://www.washingtonpost.com/wp-dyn/content/article/2009/04/26/AR2009042602711.html

[20] http://www.washingtonpost.com/wp-dyn/content/article/2009/04/26/AR2009042602711.html

[21] http://www.nytimes.com/2010/10/09/health/09drug.html

[22] http://www.redbookmag.com/health-wellness/advice/diet-pills-yl-2

[23] http://www.aneki.com/richest.html   highest GDP

[24] Wendy Chant, *Conquer the Fat-Loss Code.* : McGraw Hill, 2009. p 3-5

[25] http://health.yahoo.net/articles/nutrition/photos/7-side-effects-drinking-diet-soda#0

[26] http://health.yahoo.net/articles/nutrition/photos/7-side-effects-drinking-diet-soda#0

[27] Wendy Chant, *Conquer the Fat-Loss Code.* : McGraw Hill, 2009

[28] CNN Sanjay Gupta 91512 interview with Mayor Bloomberg

[29] http://www.nytimes.com/2012/09/14/nyregion/health-board-approves-bloombergs-soda-ban.html?_r=0

[30] http://www.fathead-movie.com/index.php/2011/09/21/interview-with-wheat-belly-author-dr-william-davis-part-two/

[31] http://www.wheatbellyblog.com/success-stories/

[32] http://well.blogs.nytimes.com/2009/07/02/celiac-disease-becoming-more-common/

[33] http://connection.ebscohost.com/c/articles/74549165/global-burden-childhood-coeliac-disease-neglected-component-diarrhoeal-mortality

[34] http://www.youtube.com/watch?v=O7ijukNzlUg

[35] http://www.nytimes.com/1990/05/08/science/huge-study-of-diet-indicts-fat-and-meat.html?pagewanted=all&src=pm

[36] http://www.medicinenet.com/script/main/art.asp?articlekey=56589

[37] http://rawfoodsos.com/2011/09/22/forks-over-knives-is-the-science-legit-a-review-and-critique/

[38] but isolated casein in rat studies is not the same as any animal protein in a real-world human diet

[39] http://rawfoodsos.com/2011/09/22/forks-over-knives-is-the-science-legit-a-review-and-critique/

[40] http://calorielab.com/restaurants/starbucks/

[41] http://www.westonaprice.org/vegetarianism-and-plant-foods/the-china-study-myth

[42] http://www.vegsource.com/news/2010/07/china-study-author-colin-campbell-slaps-down-critic-denise-minger.html

[43] http://rawfoodsos.com/2011/09/22/forks-over-knives-is-the-science-legit-a-review-and-critique/

[44] http://rawfoodsos.com/2011/09/22/forks-over-knives-is-the-science-legit-a-review-and-critique/

[45] http://rawfoodsos.com/2011/09/22/forks-over-knives-is-the-science-legit-a-review-and-critique/

[46] http://www.webmd.com/diet/pritikin-principle-what-it-is

[47] http://www.livestrong.com/article/489875-how-does-your-stomach-tell-your-brain-that-youre-full/#ixzz22EMDD9fv

[48] http://www.dailymotion.com/video/x59iwc_the-paleo-diet-and-multiple-scleros_lifestyle

[49] http://www.youtube.com/watch?v=2-VPbbu2pmU

[50] *http://en.wikipedia.org/wiki/ABO_blood_group_system*

[51] http://www.amazon.com/Eat-Right-Your-Type-Individualized/dp/039914255X

[52] http://www.dadamo.com/bloodtype_O.htm

[53] Beinfield and Korngold, *Between Heaven and Earth: A Guide to Chinese Medicine*. New York: Ballantine, 1991. p 324

[54] Beinfield and Korngold, *Between Heaven and Earth: A Guide to Chinese Medicine*. New York: Ballantine, 1991. p 325

[55] http://www.dailymail.co.uk/news/article-2083368/Former-White-House-pastry-chef-Roland-Mesnier-remembers-Bill-Clintons-big-appetite.html

[56] http://www.npr.org/blogs/thetwo-way/2012/01/09/144912442/just-how-much-did-clinton-eat-as-president

[57] http://blog.seattlepi.com/seattlepolitics/2011/08/19/bill-clinton-vegan/

[58] http://www.cnn.com/2011/HEALTH/08/18/bill.clinton.diet.vegan/index.html

[59] http://www.cbsnews.com/2100-500165_162-612689.html

[60] http://www.heart.org/idc/groups/heart-public/@wcm/@sop/@smd/documents/downloadable/ucm_319588.pdf

[61] http://www.teenhelp.com/teen-health/teen-obesity.html

[62] http://www.nytimes.com/2012/04/30/health/research/obesity-and-type-2-diabetes-cases-take-toll-on-children.html

[63] http://www.nytimes.com/2012/04/30/health/research/obesity-and-type-2-diabetes-cases-take-toll-on-children.html

[64] http://www.everydayhealth.com/family-health/kids-health/healthy-school-lunches.aspx

[65] http://www.youtube.com/watch?v=wshlnRWnf30

[66] See show at http://www.youtube.com/watch?v=wshlnRWnf30

[67] http://usnews.nbcnews.com/_news/2012/01/31/10282876-mcdonalds-drops-use-of-gooey-ammonia-based-pink-slime-in-hamburger-meat?lite

[68] http://www.cbsnews.com/8301-504763_162-57393719-10391704/report-usda-school-lunch-meat-contains-pink-slime/
[69] http://www.wanttoknow.info/050520schooldietchange
[70] http://www.organicconsumers.org/school/appleton090304.cfm
[71] http://elisabethornano-tdah.org/en/noticias/general-press/47/
[72] http://www.organicconsumers.org/school/appleton090304.cfm
[73] http://www.wholefoodsmarket.com/mission-values/environmental-stewardship/genetically-engineered-foods
[74] http://www.seattlepi.com/lifestyle/health/article/Living-Well-Blueberries-trigger-neurons-that-1153313.php#ixzz24ab89SIF
[75] http://www.seattlepi.com/lifestyle/health/article/Living-Well-Blueberries-trigger-neurons-that-1153313.php#ixzz24OrnE998
[76] http://news.nationalgeographic.com/news/2001/06/0604_wirealgae.html
[77] http://www.livestrong.com/article/200114-what-are-the-dangers-of-gmo-soybeans/#ixzz24HxXssXa
[78] http://www.independent.co.uk/news/science/gm-20-a-new-kind-of-wheat-7595087.html
[79]

https://www.google.com/search?q=Bitter+seeds%3A+the+human+toll+of+GMOs&ie=utf-8&oe=utf-8&aq=t&rls=org.mozilla:en-US:official&client=firefox-a
[80] http://www.guardian.co.uk/global-development/2012/jan/22/future-of-food-john-vidal
[81] http://www.youtube.com/watch?v=O7ijukNzlUg
[82] http://www.sustainablebusiness.com/index.cfm/go/news.feature/id/1275
[83] www.uihealthcare.com/topics/nutrition/nutr3301.html
[84] http://www.organicfooddirectory.com.au/general-issues/bioregionalism/nutrient-loss-in-transport.html
[85] http://www.guardian.co.uk/global-development/2012/jan/22/future-of-food-john-vidal Global Development is supported by the Bill and Melinda Gates Foundation
[86] http://www.foodworldnews.com/articles/1978/20120817/orange-sweet-potatoes-malnutrition-africa-vitamin-deficiency.htm
[87] http://www.youtube.com/watch?v=iwL_jw7su3U
[88] http://blog.nj.com/njv_guest_blog/2012/03/the_world_needs_new_ways_to_gr.html

[89] http://www.guardian.co.uk/global-development/2012/jan/22/future-of-food-john-vidal

[90] http://answers.yahoo.com/question/index?qid=20080919100008AApz2PK

[91] http://citygirlbites.com/blog/archives/399

[92] http://www.livestrong.com/article/315083-calories-in-a-large-movie-theater-popcorn/#ixzz23AM6KfiP

[93] http://www.livestrong.com/article/315083-calories-in-a-large-movie-theater-popcorn/#ixzz23ALhAxCL

[94] http://www.ucsusa.org/food_and_agriculture/solutions/big_picture_solutions/ensuring-the-harvest.html

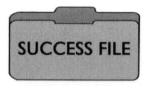

SUCCESS FILE

Success is completion * Success is deletion *Success is creation

1.	
2.	
3.	
4.	
5.	
6.	
7.	
8.	
9.	
10.	
11.	
12.	
13.	
14.	
15.	
16.	
17.	
18.	
19.	
20.	
21.	
22.	
23.	
24.	
25.	
26.	
27.	
28.	
29.	
30.	

31.	
32.	
33.	
34.	
35.	
36.	
37.	
38.	
39.	
40.	
41.	
42.	
43.	
44.	
45.	
46.	
47.	
48.	
49.	
50.	
51.	
52.	
53.	
54.	
55.	
56.	
57.	
58.	
59.	
60.	
61.	
62.	
63.	
64.	
65.	
66.	
67.	
68.	
69.	

70.	
71.	
72.	
73.	
74.	
75.	
76.	
77.	
78.	
79.	
80.	
81.	
82.	
83.	
84.	
85.	
86.	
87.	
88.	
89.	
90.	
91.	
92.	
93.	
94.	
95.	
96.	
97.	
98.	
99.	
100.	
101.	
102.	
103.	
104.	
105.	
106.	
107.	
108.	

109.	
110.	
111.	
112.	
113.	
114.	
115.	
116.	
117.	
118.	
119.	
120.	
121.	
122.	
123.	
124.	
125.	
126.	
127.	
128.	
129.	
130.	
131.	
132.	
133.	
134.	
135.	
136.	
137.	
138.	
139.	
140.	
141.	
142.	
143.	
144.	
145.	
146.	
147.	

148.	
149.	
150.	
151.	
152.	
153.	
154.	
155.	
156.	
157.	
158.	
159.	
160.	
161.	
162.	
163.	
164.	
165.	
166.	
167.	
168.	
169.	
170.	
171.	
172.	
173.	
174.	
175.	
176.	
177.	
178.	
179.	
180.	
181.	
182.	
183.	
184.	
185.	
186.	

187.	
188.	
189.	
190.	
191.	
192.	
193.	
194.	
195.	
196.	
197.	
198.	
199.	
200.	
201.	
202.	
203.	
204.	
205.	
206.	
207.	
208.	
209.	
210.	
211.	
212.	
213.	
214.	
215.	
216.	
217.	
218.	
219.	
220.	

Success is completion * Success is deletion *Success is creation

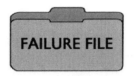

FAILURE FILE

* Failure is incompletion * Do you want to complete, delete or recreate this outcome?

1.	
2.	
3.	
4.	
5.	
6.	
7.	
8.	
9.	
10.	
11.	
12.	
13.	
14.	
15.	
16.	
17.	
18.	
19.	
20.	
21.	
22.	
23.	
24.	
25.	
26.	
27.	
28.	
29.	
30.	

31.	
32.	
33.	
34.	
35.	
36.	
37.	
38.	
39.	
40.	
41.	
42.	
43.	
44.	
45.	
46.	
47.	
48.	
49.	
50.	
51.	
52.	
53.	
54.	
55.	
56.	
57.	
58.	
59.	
60.	
61.	
62.	
63.	
64.	
65.	
66.	
67.	
68.	
69.	

70.	
71.	
72.	
73.	
74.	
75.	
76.	
77.	
78.	
79.	
80.	
81.	
82.	
83.	
84.	
85.	
86.	
87.	
88.	
89.	
90.	
91.	
92.	
93.	
94.	
95.	
96.	
97.	
98.	
99.	
100.	

Remember, failure is incompletion.

Do you want to complete, delete or recreate this now?